FAST FACTS ABOUT GI AND LIVER DISEASES FOR NURSES

D0556284

Amanda Chaney, MSN, ARNP, FNP-BC, is a liver transplant nurse practitioner, nurse practitioner advocate, and nurse leader in the nurse practitioner and transplant nursing areas. She holds an academic appointment as an assistant professor of medicine. Ms. Chaney is the author of several book chapters and articles for peer-reviewed journals and she is an avid researcher. She was chosen as one of 19 nurse practitioners from across the United States to be a part of the inaugural American Association of Nurse Practitioners (AANP) Leadership Program in 2014. To help the professional development and leadership of other nurses and nurse practitioners, she founded a group for the professional development of aspiring leaders that encourages mentorship and guides members in fine-tuning their publishing and presenting skills, while offering support and guidance for successful careers.

FAST FACTS ABOUT
GI AND LIVER DISEASES
FOR NURSES

What APRNs Need
to Know in a Nutshell

Amanda Chaney, MSN, ARNP, FNP-BC

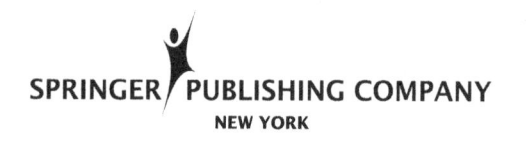

SPRINGER PUBLISHING COMPANY
NEW YORK

Springer Publishing Company, LLC
11 West 42nd Street
New York, NY 10036
www.springerpub.com

Acquisitions Editor: Margaret Zuccarini
Senior Production Editor: Kris Parrish
Compositor: S4Carlisle Publishing Services

ISBN: 978-0-8261-1724-3
e-book ISBN: 978-0-8261-1749-6

16 17 18 19 20 / 5 4 3 2 1

The author and the publisher of this Work have made every effort to use sources believed to be reliable to provide information that is accurate and compatible with the standards generally accepted at the time of publication. Because medical science is continually advancing, our knowledge base continues to expand. Therefore, as new information becomes available, changes in procedures become necessary. We recommend that the reader always consult current research and specific institutional policies before performing any clinical procedure. The author and publisher shall not be liable for any special, consequential, or exemplary damages resulting, in whole or in part, from the readers' use of, or reliance on, the information contained in this book. The publisher has no responsibility for the persistence or accuracy of URLs for external or third-party Internet websites referred to in this publication and does not guarantee that any content on such websites is, or will remain, accurate or appropriate.

Library of Congress Cataloging-in-Publication Data
Names: Chaney, Amanda, author.
Title: Fast facts about GI and liver diseases for nurses : what APRNs need to
  know in a nutshell / Amanda Chaney.
Other titles: Fast facts about gastrointestinal and liver diseases for nurses
  | Fast facts (Springer Publishing Company)
Description: New York : Springer, [2017] | Series: Fast facts | Includes
  bibliographical references and index.
Identifiers: LCCN 2016018940| ISBN 9780826117243 | ISBN 9780826117496 (e-book)
Subjects: | MESH: Gastrointestinal Diseases | Liver Diseases | Nurses'
  Instruction
Classification: LCC RC801 | NLM WI 140 | DDC 616.3/3--dc23 LC record available at https://lccn.
loc.gov/2016018940

Printed in the United States of America by Gasch Printing.

This is dedicated to my best friend, my biggest fan, and my guy, Chris. Thank you for supporting me always, no matter what.

Contents

Preface

The purpose of this book is to offer insight into the diagnosis, management, and treatment of patients with gastrointestinal (GI) and liver disease. There is not much scholarly work devoted to this topic for this select group of professionals, yet we provide a great deal of care to these patients. GI disorders and liver disease are becoming common problems in the United States, with nausea, vomiting, and abdominal pain being some of the most common complaints in the offices of primary care providers.

Each chapter provides the reader with an overview and introduction, followed by significant laboratory or imaging findings, treatment options, expected outcomes, and several "Fast Facts in a Nutshell" that will highlight key take-away points. I hope that this book will review much-needed information for those at the bedside caring for these patients, allowing more time with patients rather than fumbling through pages to find an answer on how to manage these illnesses. There is no other book in the literature that is like this one. This book offers concise information you can use to provide your patient with the best care.

Amanda Chaney

Assessment of Common Gastrointestinal Symptoms

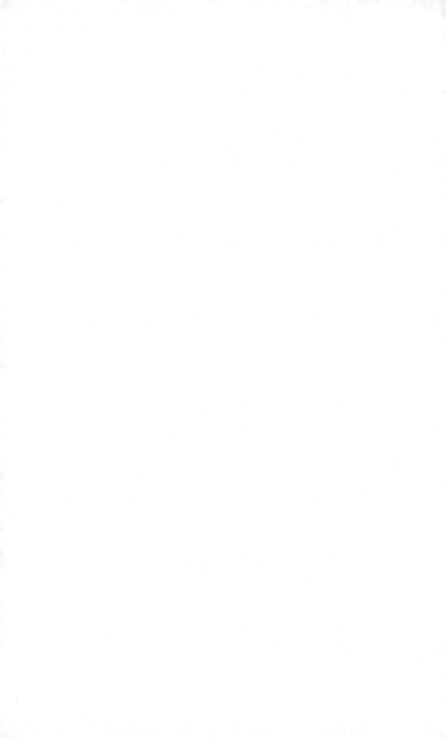

Abdominal Assessment, Labs, Imaging, and Differential Diagnosis

The gastrointestinal (GI) system is a very complex and multifaceted system. It encompasses not only the GI tract, including the esophagus, stomach, and the small and large bowel (or luminal GI), but also the salivary glands, liver, biliary system and gallbladder, and pancreas (or the hepato-biliary-pancreatic GI; Chang & Leung, 2014). These organs are responsible for aiding the body in fuel consumption and nutrition, as well as in providing blood-clotting factors and supporting immunity. The abdominal assessment is an essential tool for providers to diagnose and treat GI illnesses appropriately.

At the end of this chapter, the reader will be able to:

1. Name two history questions that are important for a thorough abdominal assessment
2. Describe when ordering specific abdominal imaging is necessary
3. State the proper order of the physical exam for the abdomen

Good assessment skills begin with taking a thorough patient history. A thorough history must include a diet history, presence of abdominal distension or bloating, nausea, vomiting, diarrhea, constipation, number of bowel movements per day, characteristics and color of bowel movements, blood in vomit (hematemesis), bright-red blood from the rectum (or hematochezia), black and/or tarry stools (melena), alternating patterns of diarrhea and constipation, presence of reflux, or trouble tolerating certain foods. It is also important to discuss any associated symptoms that are occurring, such as fever, chills, shortness of breath, or yellowing of skin or sclera.

Once a thorough history is obtained, the provider should perform a complete abdominal examination (Table 1.1).

First, ensure the patient is lying down comfortably and that privacy is protected. Inspection is the first part of the abdominal examination. One must evaluate for any masses, nodules, superficial veins, or hernias. Look at the patient's skin and note whether there is any discoloration, rashes, scars, or any other lesions (Cox & Stegall, 2009). In particularly thin individuals, one may see pulsations of the aorta.

Next, the provider should auscultate the abdomen. The order of this step is particularly important, as palpation and percussion can stimulate bowel motility and give a false impression of true bowel sounds and function. The provider should auscultate the abdomen using a systematic approach, moving through each abdominal quadrant (right upper quadrant [RUQ], left upper quadrant [LUQ], right lower quadrant [RLQ], and left lower quadrant [LLQ]). Bowel sounds should be noted for quality (high- or low-pitched)and frequency (hyperactive versus

---

TABLE 1.1 The Abdominal Examination Process

1. Inspection
2. Auscultation
3. Percussion
4. Palpation

hypoactive versus absent). Listen for other sounds as well, such as pulsations or bruits, which could be indicative of a vascular issue (e.g., aneurysm or vascular stenosis; Cox & Stegall, 2009).

Percussion, followed by palpation, is next in the abdominal examination. Percussing the four quadrants can be helpful in distinguishing fluid (dull sounds) versus air (high-pitched sounds) in the abdomen. Gentle palpation should be performed systematically through the four quadrants, followed by deep palpation. Any pain, tenderness, or guarding should be noted, as well as whether the edges of the spleen and/or liver are felt (Cox & Stegall, 2009).

The final step is the digital rectal examination, which should be performed in all patients with abdominal/rectal pain and/or if gastrointestinal bleeding is suspected (Goff, 2015).

If there is a concern about appendicitis, the iliopsoas and obturator tests can be performed. In the iliopsoas test, the patient is supine and asked to raise one leg at a time. If the patient has right lower abdominal pain, it means there is inflammation of the right psoas muscle. This could be an indication of appendicitis. In the obturator test, the patient's thigh is flexed at a 90° angle and rotated outward. If there is pain with this movement, possible causes are appendicitis or abscess of the right ovary or fallopian tube (Goff, 2015).

A positive Murphy's sign is present when the patient stops breathing with palpation of the right upper quadrant (Goff, 2015).

PERTINENT LABORATORY FINDINGS

Routine blood work, including complete blood count to rule out anemia or infection (hemoglobin and hematocrit [H&H] and white blood count [WBC]), complete metabolic panel (evaluating for electrolyte imbalances and renal function), urinalysis, and (if pancreatitis is suspected) amylase and lipase tests are useful. Liver function tests* can be helpful in determining whether there are biliary or hepatic diseases. A stool test for occult blood is recommended if there is concern about GI bleeding or if the patient has anemia. (Goff, 2015).

*For further discussion on abnormal liver function tests (LFTs), see Chapter 15.

All women of childbearing age should have a pregnancy test (beta human chorionic gonadotropin test; Goff, 2015).

IMAGING/DIAGNOSTIC STUDIES

- Plain flat/upright abdominal films: These are least expensive and readily available. These films can detect an ileus, a bowel obstruction, or perforation of the bowel (Goff, 2015).
- Abdominal ultrasound: Noninvasive; can be done at the bedside. Abnormalities of the gallbladder, pelvic organs, appendix, kidneys, and liver can be determined by ultrasound. A complete examination may be difficult in patients with a large abdominal girth (Goff, 2015).
- CT: A useful and frequently ordered test when trying to determine cause of acute abdominal pain (Goff, 2015). Contrast is given usually both orally (better evaluation of gastrointestinal tract) and intravenously (better evaluation of vasculature).
- MRI: Expensive and usually not indicated in the acute setting. It is useful when evaluating for hepatocellular carcinoma and metastatic disease; used to better evaluate lesion(s) seen on CT scan.
- Hepatobiliary iminodiacetic acid (HIDA) scan: This is a beneficial test when ruling out acute cholecystitis (Goff, 2015).
- Esophagogastroduodenoscopy (EGD): A procedure performed by a gastroenterologist to evaluate the upper structures of the GI tract.
- Colonoscopy: A procedure performed by a gastroenterologist to evaluate the large intestine and rectum.

For a generalized list of differential diagnoses that are possible for GI diseases, see Table 1.2.

ICD-10 CODE

Abnormal bowel sounds: R19.15
Absent bowel: R19.11
Change in bowel habit: R19.4
Hyperactive bowel sounds: R19.12

TABLE 1.2 Gastrointestinal Issues

Acute appendicitis	Inflammatory bowel disease
Acute pancreatitis	(Crohn's disease or ulcerative
Cirrhosis	colitis)
Gastroenteritis	Viral hepatitis
Peritonitis	Celiac disease
GI cancers (gastric, colorectal,	Food intolerances
hepatocellular)	Peptic ulcers
Irritable bowel syndrome	Diverticulitis
Acute liver failure	Gallstones, acute cholecystitis
Pregnancy/miscarriage	Ectopic pregnancy

GI, gastrointestinal.

════════════════ FAST FACTS in a NUTSHELL

1. Remember the proper order of the abdominal examination: inspection, auscultation, percussion, palpation.
2. Perform a thorough history to formulate the differential diagnosis. Don't be afraid to get "too personal"—especially about bowel movements. It is important not to miss information about black or bloody stools.
3. Plain x-rays are very useful when evaluating the patient with GI issues. It may not be necessary to jump right to ordering a CT scan. Remember, CT scans come with a financial cost and deliver much more radiation than plain abdominal films.

REFERENCES

Chang, E. B., & Leung, P. S. (2014). Regulation of gastrointestinal functions. In P. S. Leung (Ed.), *The gastrointestinal system: Gastrointestinal, nutritional and hepatobiliary physiology* (pp. 3–34). Dordrecht, Netherlands: Springer Science.

Cox, C., & Stegall, M. (2009). A step-by-step guide to performing a complete abdominal examination. *Gastrointestinal Nursing, 7*(1), 10–17.

Goff, J. S. (2015). Evaluation of acute abdominal pain. In P. R. McNally (Ed.), *GI/liver secrets plus* (5th ed., pp. 398–404). Philadelphia, PA: Elsevier Saunders.

2

Nausea and Vomiting

*Nausea and vomiting can come without warning and can
be attributed to a variety of causes. There are several key
diagnoses not to be missed when this occurs (Goroll & Mulley,
2014). In normal gastrointestinal (GI) function, there is a
communication between the brain and the GI tract. Nausea
usually occurs prior to vomiting, which is a bodily response
to remove toxins. Certain neurotransmitters are responsible
for controlling the vomiting reflex (Longstreth, 2015).*

At the end of this chapter, the reader will be able to:

1. Identify three not-to-miss diagnoses associated with nausea and vomiting
2. Name three classes of medications used to treat nausea and vomiting
3. State two risk factors associated with nausea and vomiting

INCIDENCE

Nausea and vomiting (N/V) are common complaints (2%) in primary care offices. Their economic burden reaches $4 to 10 billion annually in the United States (Goroll & Mulley, 2014).

ASSESSMENT

Initial evaluation of the patient with nausea and vomiting includes determining how long the patient has had symptoms. If longer than 1 month, the patient is considered to have chronic symptoms (Longstreth, 2015). A careful history should include questions regarding the patient's food history, recent travel, recent exposure to sick individuals, and change in or addition of new medications. The patient should be asked about any associated symptoms (i.e., fever, chills, chest pain, abdominal pain, abdominal distension, etc.). The provider should document the frequency of vomiting episodes as well as characteristics of the emesis (Longstreth, 2015).

The most common complications of nausea and vomiting are dehydration and conditions caused by electrolyte imbalances, mainly hypokalemia and metabolic alkalosis (Longstreth, 2015). Very young patients and the elderly are at particularly high risk for developing dehydration, so careful attention to these patients is important.

Physical examination should include vital signs with careful attention to blood pressure and heart rate (hypotension and tachycardia can be signs of severe dehydration). The provider should perform a thorough abdominal examination, noting bowel sounds, abdominal distension and/or tenderness/pain, and other associated symptoms (American Gastroenterological Association, 2001).

PERTINENT LABORATORY FINDINGS

Depending on the degree of dehydration, basic laboratory evaluation may be needed to evaluate specifically for anemia, infection, and electrolyte imbalances. Studies can include complete blood count and complete metabolic panel. For women of childbearing age, a pregnancy test should be obtained. Other tests based on history can be requested including thyroid studies and therapeutic drug studies (e.g., digoxin levels; American Gastroenterological Association, 2001).

When concerned about an infectious cause, stool samples can be sent for analysis for causes of acute nausea and vomiting (Longstreth, 2015).

ADDITIONAL STUDIES

Esophagogastroduodenoscopy (EGD) can be performed for patients with unexplained nausea and vomiting (chronic; Longstreth, 2015).

Abdominal x-rays can be performed if there is concern about a bowel obstruction (American Gastroenterological Association, 2001).

DIFFERENTIAL DIAGNOSIS

- Life-threatening disorders (Longstreth, 2015)
  - Myocardial infarction
  - Bowel obstruction
  - Mesenteric ischemia
  - Acute pancreatitis
- Cholelithiasis (associated with abdominal pain; Longstreth, 2015)
- Gastroesophageal reflux disease (GERD)—chronic nausea (Longstreth, 2015)
- Vertigo, vestibular neuritis (Longstreth, 2015)
- Metabolic causes—diabetic ketoacidosis, Addisonian crisis, uremia, hyponatremia, binge drinkers (Goroll & Mulley, 2014)
- Early pregnancy (Goroll & Mulley, 2014; Longstreth, 2015)
- Functional N/V (Goroll & Mulley, 2014)
- Peptic ulcer disease and gastritis—usually postprandial emesis; coffee-ground emesis (more serious and can lead to severe anemia—a life-threatening issue); patient may have nausea with a bad taste in the mouth in the morning (Goroll & Mulley, 2014)
- Gastroparesis—gastric distension caused by food retained in the stomach for more than 6 hours after eating; can occur in patients with diabetes (Goroll & Mulley, 2014; Longstreth, 2015)

- Acute gastroenteritis—most likely a viral cause, such as rotavirus, norovirus, and enteric adenovirus (Longstreth, 2015):
  - Nausea, vomiting, diarrhea, cramping abdominal pain, myalgias, headache, and fever
  - Quick recovery, but symptoms can last for 7 to 10 days (Goroll & Mulley, 2014)
- Neurologic emergencies (Goroll & Mulley, 2014)
  - Midline cerebellar hemorrhage—nausea and vomiting are profuse and associated with severe gait ataxia, meningeal signs, and headache; can be fatal
  - Increased intracranial pressure—one third will have vomiting
- Migraine headache (Goroll & Mulley, 2014; Longstreth, 2015)
- Drugs—digitalis toxicity, chemotherapy (Goroll & Mulley, 2014; Longstreth, 2015)
- Postoperative—usually a side effect of general anesthesia (Longstreth, 2015)
- Psychiatric disorders, including depression, anxiety, bulimia nervosa, or anorexia nervosa (American Gastroenterological Association, 2001)

TREATMENT OPTIONS

For patients who are dehydrated, intravenous fluids (IVFs) are usually needed to assist with hydration until oral intake is possible. Providers usually choose normal saline with potassium to supplement fluid losses (American Gastroenterological Association, 2001).

Here are the most common medication choices used to control nausea and vomiting:

- Antiemetics—medications that work by controlling response from the central nervous system (Hasler & Chey, 2003):
  - Ondansetron (Zofran): Common side effect is constipation (Hasler & Chey, 2003).
  - Prochlorperazine (Phenergan): Side effects include hypotension and sedating properties. Should be used with

caution in patients with neurological issues, the elderly, or patients with liver disease (Longstreth, 2015).

- Prokinetics—alter the motility of the GI tract (Hasler & Chey, 2003):
  - Metoclopramide (Reglan): Considered a dopamine receptor antagonist; side effects include extrapyramidal effects. Cautious use required in patients with neurological issues and in elderly patients (Longstreth, 2015).

For chronic conditions, alternative therapies, such as acupuncture, biofeedback, meditation, and psychotherapy, have proven to be effective (Hasler & Chey, 2003).

ICD-10 CODE

Nausea: R11.0
Nausea with vomiting, unspecified: R11.2
Vomiting without nausea: R11.11

======= *FAST FACTS in a NUTSHELL*

1. Nausea and vomiting are common medical problems in primary care and can be attributed to mild acute gastroenteritis, to more serious and life-threatening issues such as intracranial bleeding or myocardial infarction.
2. A thorough history is needed to identify the cause of nausea and vomiting so as not to miss conditions that require emergent care.
3. The key to management is symptom control and avoiding dehydration and electrolyte imbalances.

REFERENCES

American Gastroenterological Association. (2001). American Gastroenterological Association medical position statement: Nausea and vomiting. *Gastroenterology, 120,* 263–286.

Goroll, A. H., & Mulley, A. G. (2014). *Primary care medicine: Office evaluation and management of the adult patient* (7th ed., pp. 459–628). Philadelphia, PA: Lippincott Williams & Wilkins.

Hasler, W. L., & Chey, W. D. (2003). Nausea and vomiting. *Gastroenterology, 125*, 1860–1867. doi:10.1053/j.gastro.2003.09.040

Longstreth, G. F. (2015). Approach to the adult with nausea and vomiting. Retrieved from www.uptodate.com/contents/approach-to-the-adult-with-nausea-and-vomiting?source=search_result&search=nausea+and+vomiting&selectedTitle=1%7E150.html

3

Abdominal Pain

Abdominal pain can occur in a patient for any number of reasons (see Differential Diagnosis section). The key for providers is to determine whether the abdominal pain is life threatening and, if so, to get the patient the proper medical care.

At the end of this chapter, the reader will be able to:

1. Define the *surgical* or *acute abdomen*
2. Name two causes of acute abdominal pain
3. State four questions that should be asked when obtaining a history of the patient with abdominal pain

ASSESSMENT

When evaluating the patient with abdominal pain, obtaining a detailed history is important in determining the proper diagnosis. First of all, a description of the abdominal pain is necessary; key descriptors are terms such as *dull, aching, sharp,* and *colicky.* Providers should ask when the pain started; how long he or she has had pain; where it started; whether this kind

TABLE 3.1 Red Flags of Abdominal Assessment

Fever	Abdominal pain with movement* (peritonitis)
Tachycardia	Third spacing or edema
Tachypnea	Scleral icterus
Hypotension	Jaundice
Rebound tenderness	Abnormal bowel sounds (absent or hyperactive)
Tympany, on percussion	
Guarding, muscular rigidity, or spasm with palpation* (peritonitis)	Presence of friction rub on abdominal auscultation
Board-like abdomen*	Leukocytosis

*Peritoneal signs.
Adapted from Fishman and Aronson (2013) and Rothchild and Schoen (2015).

of pain occurred before; how often the pain occurs; whether the pain moves or radiates to another part of the body; whether pain starts or stops in relation to food intake; and whether there are other aggravating and alleviating factors and any other accompanying symptoms, such as fever, chills, nausea, vomiting, abdominal distension, or blood in emesis or stools (Fishman & Aronson, 2013; Goff, 2015; Penner & Majumdar, 2013). Women of childbearing age should be asked about their menstrual history and the possibility of pregnancy (Fishman & Aronson, 2013). Medical history should be reviewed; if patient has a history of diabetes, chronic renal failure, is immunosuppressed, or uses steroids (Goff, 2015), it should be noted. It is also important to be aware of the patient's prior surgical history, as some patients may have chronic abdominal pain because of adhesions and scar tissue (Rothchild & Schoen, 2015).

A thorough physical examination should be performed. Vital signs should be obtained and a detailed abdominal examination including a rectal examination, and pelvic examination (for women), should be performed (Table 3.1; Fishman & Aronson, 2013; Goff, 2015). See Chapter 1 for details on abdominal examination.

PERTINENT LABORATORY FINDINGS

In the patient with acute abdominal pain, laboratory testing should include complete blood count with differential, complete metabolic panel, lipase and amylase tests, liver function tests, urinalysis, and pregnancy test (for premenopausal women). Blood and urine cultures should be obtained if the patient is febrile or appears ill/unstable (Goff, 2015; Penner & Majumdar, 2013).

Stool samples for occult blood should be obtained.

IMAGING STUDIES

Abdominal flat and upright films are useful in the patient presenting with abdominal pain. Bowel obstruction or intestinal perforation can be seen on these films. If CT scan is available, it is the preferred first imaging study for patients with a more urgent presentation. Abdominal ultrasound imaging is preferred in those cases in which peritonitis is a concern and/or if the patient is pregnant or possibly pregnant (Penner & Majumdar, 2013).

DIFFERENTIAL DIAGNOSIS

- "Surgical abdomen" or an "acute abdomen"—are terms used to describe abdominal pain that quickly worsens and will likely continue to do so without surgery; considered in cases of infarction, bowel obstruction, and peritonitis (Goff, 2015; Penner & Majumdar, 2013)
- Obstruction—described as a colicky, wavelike pain; can develop over days to months
  - Symptoms: colicky pain from beginning; nausea with vomiting; distended abdomen; no bowel movements for a day to several days, constipation, or diarrhea (Goroll & Mulley, 2014; Penner & Majumdar, 2013)
  - Examination: high-pitched hyperactive or no bowel sounds; tympanic sounds on percussion; may test positive for occult blood (Goroll & Mulley, 2014; Penner & Majumdar, 2013)
  - Abdominal films: distension of loops of bowel with high air–fluid levels (Goroll & Mulley, 2014; Penner & Majumdar, 2013)

- Peritonitis
  - Symptoms: unable to lie still; fever, chills, nausea, vomiting (Goroll & Mulley, 2014; Penner & Majumdar, 2013)
  - Examination: rebound tenderness; positive psoas sign; hypoactive bowel sounds; abdominal muscle stiffness (Goroll & Mulley, 2014; Penner & Majumdar, 2013)
- Acute appendicitis
  - Gradual pain that worsens over hours (Goff, 2015)
  - Associated with anorexia, nausea, vomiting, fever (Goff, 2015)
- Aortic dissection or aortic aneurysm rupture (requires immediate surgical intervention)
  - Presents with severe acute abdominal pain that radiates to back or genitalia (Goroll & Mulley, 2014; Penner & Majumdar, 2013)
  - May have pulsatile, painful abdominal mass; abdominal bruit may or may not be present (Goroll & Mulley, 2014; Penner & Majumdar, 2013)
- Mesenteric ischemia or infarction
  - Pain usually out of proportion with physical examination; requires surgical intervention (Penner & Majumdar, 2013; Rothchild & Schoen, 2015)
  - Consider in patients who have thromboembolic history or clotting disorder, recent atrial fibrillation, or in those patients who are illicit drug users (aka "crack belly"; Goff, 2015; Rothchild & Schoen, 2015)
- Biliary obstruction
  - Cystic duct: also called biliary colic (passage of gallstone); sudden-onset severe pain, usually lasting 1 hour; typically in the right upper quadrant (RUQ), or epigastric pain that radiates to the scapular area; associated symptoms may include nausea, vomiting, fever, positive Murphy's sign (Goff, 2015; Goroll & Mulley, 2014; Penner & Majumdar, 2013)
  - Common bile duct: pain usually in the epigastric area; nausea, vomiting, jaundice; tenderness in RUQ; if associated with weight loss, consider malignancy (liver or biliary; Goroll & Mulley, 2014; Penner & Majumdar, 2013)
- Acute cholecystitis
  - Patient may have a history of prior episodes of abdominal pain; pain occurs after a meal, particularly after a fatty

meal and at night; pain increases over 20 to 30 minutes, moves to the back and/or scapula, then improves; may have nausea, vomiting, and fever; may have positive Murphy's sign (Goff, 2015)
- Ascending cholangitis
  - Presents with fever, jaundice, RUQ abdominal pain (Penner & Majumdar, 2013)
  - May have abnormal liver function, particularly elevated bilirubin levels
  - Requires prompt identification and treatment, as these patients can quickly develop sepsis and septic shock
  - May need endoscopic retrograde cholangiopancreatography (ERCP) if concerned with biliary strictures as a cause of cholangitis
- Pancreatitis
  - Acute: presents with constant epigastric pain, periumbilical, or left or right upper abdominal pain radiating to back (classic presentation); pain sometimes is increased with food intake; associated symptoms can include nausea, vomiting, lack of appetite (anorexia), fever; distended abdomen; decreased bowel sounds; often associated with a gallstone complication; alcohol intake, recent ERCP procedure, and recent trauma are risk factors; elevated lipase in combination with epigastric pain suggests pancreatitis (Goroll & Mulley, 2014; Penner & Majumdar, 2013)
  - Chronic: intermittent episodes of epigastric pain, often after alcohol consumption; risk factor—alcoholic patients (Goroll & Mulley, 2014; Penner & Majumdar, 2013)
- Lower abdominal pain (Goroll & Mulley, 2014; Penner & Majumdar, 2013)
  - Inflammatory bowel disease (IBD)—Crohn's disease or ulcerative colitis
  - Colitis
  - Renal colic (flank pain that radiates to the groin); sudden onset of pain and cramping; acute pyelonephritis: upper abdominal and/or back pain, fever and chills, urgency, dysuria
  - Female patients: pelvic inflammatory disease (PID), ectopic pregnancy, endometriosis, fallopian tube/ovarian rupture or torsion

- Diverticulitis
  - Presents in patients 50 years or older; left lower quadrant abdominal pain; mass noted on left lower quadrant on palpation; may have leukocytosis (elevated white cell count) and fever (Goff, 2015)
- Peptic ulcer disease
  - Presents with epigastric pain; described as gnawing, aching, and burning pain; pain radiating to the back suggests perforation into the pancreas (Goroll & Mulley, 2014).

ICD-10 CODE

Abdominal pain, unspecified: R10.9
Acute abdomen: R10.0

FAST FACTS in a NUTSHELL

1. Providers should be aware of signs or "red flags" in patients with abdominal pain that require immediate referral to an emergency room.
2. A referral for an expert opinion is recommended in those patients requiring an invasive procedure, who have abdominal pain lasting for more than 2 to 3 months, patients with significant unintended weight loss, jaundice, or anemia issues.
3. Rectal and pelvic examinations are necessary for those patients who present with abdominal pain.
4. Obtain a thorough history to narrow possible differential diagnoses.

REFERENCES

Goff, J. S. (2015). Evaluation of acute abdominal pain. In P. R. McNally (Ed.), *GI/liver secrets plus* (5th ed., pp. 398–404). Philadelphia, PA: Elsevier Saunders.

Goroll, A. H., & Mulley, A. G. (2014). *Primary care medicine: Office evaluation and management of the adult patient* (7th ed., pp. 459–628). Philadelphia, PA: Lippincott Williams & Wilkins.

Penner, R. M., Fishman, M. B., & Majumdar, S. R. (2016). Evaluation of the adult with abdominal pain. Retrieved from www.uptodate.com/contents/evaluation-of-the-adult-with-abdominal-pain?source=search_result&search=abdominal+pain&selectedTitle=1%7E150#H29.html

Rothchild, K., & Schoen, J. A. (2015). Surgical approach to the acute abdomen. In P. R. McNally (Ed.), *GI/liver secrets plus* (5th ed., pp. 609–613). Philadelphia, PA: Elsevier Saunders.

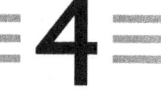

Constipation

> Constipation is defined as bowel movements that are infrequent; it is characterized by hardened stool that is difficult to evacuate. Most people have three to five bowel movements (BMs) per week, although this can vary greatly individually (Goroll & Mulley, 2014). Most providers define constipation as infrequent bowel movements of less than three per week; however, patients usually provide a wide variety of additional complaints, including straining to evacuate stool; abdominal distension and bloating; passage of hard, pellet-like stools; and even the need to manually disimpact stools (American Gastroenterological Association, 2013).

At the end of this chapter, the reader will be able to:

1. Identify three history questions that should be asked when gathering information on the patient with constipation
2. State a physical examination finding the patient with constipation may have that requires immediate attention
3. State two treatments that can be recommended initially to manage constipation

INCIDENCE AND RISK FACTORS

Constipation is common, affecting 15% of adults in Western countries and 33% of patients older than 60 (American Gastroenterological Association, 2013; Goroll & Mullen, 2014; Roque & Bouras, 2015). Frequently, patients with constipation look to self-medicate with over-the-counter remedies (Goroll & Mullen, 2014). Elderly patients have a high prevalence of laxative use; up to 74% of nursing home residents (Roque & Bouras, 2015) use laxatives daily.

ASSESSMENT

A thorough history is important when trying to determine the cause of constipation. The patient should be asked for a detailed description of bowel movements, including how many per day or week, how often, and how long has constipation been a problem. Other details include a review of all medications, including all over-the-counter, herbal, and prescription medications; use of fiber or laxatives; and review of dietary intake, including the amount of fruits and vegetables consumed. The provider should ask about the presence of associated symptoms (abdominal pain, gas, bloating, rectal bleeding, fever, cramping, vomiting, weight loss, melena, rectal pain, anorexia, mucus in stool, headache, depression, anxiety; Goroll & Mullen, 2014).

On examination, the patient's weight should be recorded and recent weight loss or gain noted. A complete abdominal examination is required. Providers should evaluate for abdominal masses, distension, tenderness, high-pitched or absent bowel sounds, rectal examination, fissures, inflammation of rectal area, and hard stool. Documentation of stool color and fecal occult blood test should be included (Goroll & Mullen, 2014).

PERTINENT LABORATORY/IMAGING TESTING

A complete blood count and complete metabolic panel should be obtained (American Gastroenterological Association, 2013).

Several electrolyte imbalances can cause constipation. Also, diabetes can cause gastroparesis and hypothyroidism can slow down gastrointestinal (GI) motility, so a measurement of glucose levels and thyroid studies may be helpful (Goroll & Mullen, 2014).

Abdominal x-rays can be obtained if there is a concern regarding bowel obstruction (Goroll & Mullen, 2014).

Colonoscopy, CT scan, flexible sigmoidoscopy, and/or barium enema can be considered if additional studies are warranted (American Gastroenterological Association, 2013; Goroll & Mullen, 2014).

DIFFERENTIAL DIAGNOSIS

Constipation is often caused by inadequate fiber intake or hydration, inactivity, or can be medication related. Other more serious causes could be obstruction, motor dysfunction as with irritable bowel syndrome (IBS), electrolyte imbalances (hypokalemia and hypercalcemia), hypothyroidism, neurologic disorders (Parkinson's disease), colorectal cancer, anal fissures or strictures, and pelvic floor dysfunction. Certain medications that can cause constipation include anticholinergic medications, codeine cough suppressants, narcotics, iron supplements, and calcium antacids (American Gastroenterological Association, 2013; Goroll & Mullen, 2014).

TREATMENT OPTIONS

After careful review of current medications and medications that may cause constipation have been identified, discontinuation of those medications may correct the problem.

Providers should encourage patients with acute constipation to increase hydration and fiber intake to 20 to 35 grams per day (Wald, 2015). Nutritional modification may be enough to resolve constipation and will likely prevent further episodes. Over-the-counter laxatives can be recommended for short-term treatment (Table 4.1). Prescription options to

TABLE 4.1 Over-the-Counter Recommendations for Management of Constipation

Osmotic agents —Synthetic disaccharides	Milk of Magnesia 1 oz by mouth twice a day Polyethylene glycol 17 g by mouth daily Lactulose 15 mL once a day
Stimulant laxative	Bisacodyl suppository via rectum once a day Glycerol suppository via rectum once a day
Fiber/bulk-forming laxatives	Psyllium 1 tbsp by mouth one to three times per day Methylcellulose 1 tbsp one to three times per day
Stool softeners	Docusate sodium 100 mg once or twice per day

Adapted from the American Gastroenterological Association (2013) and Wald (2015).

manage chronic constipation are lubiprostone and linaclotide. If patient continues to have issues after initial recommendations are completed, he or she should call the provider and return to the clinic (American Gastroenterological Association, 2013; Goroll & Mullen, 2014; Wald, 2015). If chronic constipation is or becomes an issue, referral to a specialist is recommended.

In some cases of chronic constipation, nonpharmacologic treatments are helpful. Biofeedback and relaxation techniques have been shown to provide relief in more than half of patients with structural issues and pelvic floor disorders (American Gastroenterological Association, 2013).

ICD-10 CODE

Other constipation: K59.09
Constipation, unspecified: K59.00
Outlet dysfunction constipation: K59.02
Slow transit constipation: K59.01

1. Constipation can be a symptom of some other problem (i.e., metabolic or neurologic disorder).
2. Dietary modifications are usually the most helpful way to treat constipation and prevent further episodes.
3. Over-the-counter laxatives can be recommended for safe and effective treatment of constipation for short-term therapy.

REFERENCES

American Gastroenterological Association. (2013). American Gastro-enterological Association medical position statement on constipation. *Gastroenterology, 144*, 211–217.

Goroll, A. H., & Mulley, A. G. (2014). *Primary care medicine: Office evaluation and management of the adult patient* (7th ed., pp. 459–628). Philadelphia, PA: Lippincott Williams & Wilkins.

Roque, M. V., & Bouras, E. P. (2015). Epidemiology and management of chronic constipation in elderly patients. *Clinical Interventions in Aging, 10*, 919–930. doi:10.2147/CIA.S54304

Wald, A. (2015). Management of chronic constipation in adults. Retrieved from www.uptodate.com/contents/management-of-chronic-constipation-in-adults?source=search_result&search=Management+of+chronic+constipation+in+adults.&selectedTitle=1%7E150

5

Diarrhea

Diarrhea can be further classified into acute versus chronic. Acute diarrhea is defined as loose stools that have lasted no longer than 2 weeks (Goroll & Mulley, 2014). Chronic diarrhea is defined as loose stools, or reduced stool consistency, that has lasted longer than 4 weeks (Bonis & Lamont, 2015).

At the end of this chapter, the reader will be able to:

1. Differentiate between acute and chronic diarrhea
2. Name three reasons why a patient would have chronic diarrhea
3. State three nutritional modifications that are recommended to minimize risk of dehydration

INCIDENCE AND RISK FACTORS

Diarrheal diseases are one of the top leading causes of death worldwide (Wanke, 2015). Although in normal healthy people diarrhea is considered a self-limiting illness, certain individuals can be susceptible to severe dehydration that can cause serious complications. Bacterial causes of diarrhea typically cause more severe episodes (Wanke, 2015). According to the Centers for Disease Control (CDC), approximately 48 million Americans become ill from a foodborne illness every year, 128,000 of whom are hospitalized, and 3,000 of whom die (CDC, 2015). Patients at highest risk for complications from diarrheal illnesses are individuals who are very young (infants), elderly, and/or immunocompromised. Attending or working in a day care center, travel to developing countries, and /or individuals who take or who have taken antibiotics recently are also at high risk for diarrheal illnesses (Gutierrez, Campbell, Cunningham, Riddle, & Young, 2015).

ASSESSMENT FINDINGS

When obtaining a history from the patient with diarrhea, several questions must be asked. Providers should ask about the patient's definition of *diarrhea,* as individuals may differ on its meaning. Providers should ask about occupational exposure, recent travel history, any association with bowel movements, and food consumption. Poor food-preparation techniques can be the cause of some food-borne illnesses. This can be discussed with the patient to determine whether poor technique is to blame for diarrheal illness. Specifics are noted on recent (past 24 hours) dietary history, as well as recent weight loss (intended or unintended). Review of current medications, as well as discussion of recent changes in medications, is important. Providers must question whether the patient has had recent surgery or hospitalizations, recent antibiotic use, or if there has been recent contact with sick people (others with similar symptoms). Patient should report the nature of bowel movements, including description of stool (color, notation of bloody and/or mucus; consistency; and frequency), how often bowel movements occur, and any associated symptoms (fever, nausea, vomiting, myalgia, headache, cramps, severe abdominal pain, fecal incontinence, or tenesmus; Goroll & Mulley, 2014; Wanke, 2015).

Physical examination is focused on determining the patient's hydration status. Vital signs are obtained and noted, with careful attention if there is a temperature (> 38.5 °C/101.3 °F), tachycardia, or hypotension, as these could be signs of sepsis and/or severe dehydration. Weight loss is noted. It is important to examine the skin for dryness, turgor, and to assess the patient's mucous membranes (dry versus moist) to evaluate for dehydration. A full abdominal examination is done, noting abdominal tenderness or pain, bowel sound characteristics, or any masses or abdominal bloating/fullness. Note presence of rash or "rose spots." If stool specimen is available, examine the stool characteristics, including color, consistency, and noting the presence of blood or mucus (Goroll & Mulley, 2014). Signs of inflammation and more serious illness are blood in the stool, fever, signs of hypovolemia, and severe abdominal pain (Wanke, 2015).

PERTINENT LABORATORY FINDINGS

Obtain complete blood count (CBC) and chemistry panel (looking for electrolyte imbalances). Stool specimen is obtained and sent to test for leukocytes or lactoferrin (presence of lactoferrin shows inflammation and is a marker of leukocytes). Stool cultures are usually not recommended as diarrhea is a self-limiting disease (Goroll & Mulley, 2014). Cultures are recommended, however, in patients who have inflammatory bowel disease and who are immunocompromised, have severe, inflammatory diarrhea, or have bloody diarrhea (Wanke, 2015).

If diarrhea has been ongoing for 2 or more weeks, send stool specimen for blood, ova, and parasites (if giardiasis is suspected, three specimens are needed for confirmation). If diarrhea has been ongoing for 4 weeks or more, seek consultation with an expert (Goroll & Mulley, 2014).

DIFFERENTIAL DIAGNOSIS

- Acute diarrhea—duration less than 2 weeks
  - Acute gastroenteritis (Goroll & Mulley, 2014)
    - Viral: Most commonly caused by noroviruses, such as rotavirus. Symptoms last 1 week with an incubation

period of 48 to 72 hours. Symptoms include diarrhea, nausea, vomiting, headache, low-grade fever, abdominal cramps, and malaise. The illness is self-limiting in most cases, with resolution of symptoms after 24 to 96 hours.

- Bacterial (Goroll & Mulley, 2014; Gutierrez et al., 2015)
  - *Staphylococcus aureus*: caused by a contaminant in custard-filled pastries and processed meats. Symptoms include nausea, vomiting, abdominal cramps, diarrhea within 2 to 8 hours of ingestion; usually self-limiting, with resolution of symptoms in 12 hours.
  - *Clostridium perfringens**: food contaminant; bacteria releases endotoxin in the intestine. Incubation period of eight to 24 hours. Symptoms include diarrhea, abdominal cramps, and sometimes vomiting.
  - *Bacillus cereus*: releases an endotoxin found in rice. Symptoms include severe cramping and diarrhea; incubation is 8 to 16 hours.
  - *Escherichia coli* 0157:H7: responsible for 2.5% of all cases of acute diarrhea. Caused by ingestion of contaminated meat, unpasteurized juices, fruits, and vegetables; toxins can cause mucosal edema, ulceration, and hemorrhage. Incubation time is 3 days. Symptoms range from mild, crampy diarrhea to potentially fatal hemorrhagic colitis complicated by hemolytic-uremic syndrome or thrombotic thrombocytopenic purpura.
  - Salmonella*: bacteria invade the bowel wall. Mostly likely caused by contaminated eggs or poultry. Incubation period is 12 to 36 hours and lasts approximately 2 weeks. Causes watery diarrhea, abdominal cramps, nausea, vomiting, and fever.
    - ○ Typhoid fever: **It is rare but do not miss** *Salmonella typhi*. Classic form is "pea-soup" diarrhea that starts in the third week of illness. Symptoms include a progressive fever, bradycardia, temporary rash on trunk ("rose spots"), splenomegaly, cough, headache,

---

*Most common according to the CDC (2015).

and right lower quadrant abdominal pain. Stool shows mononuclear leukocyte cells.

– *Clostridium difficile* infection/pseudomembranous colitis (Goroll & Mulley, 2014)

  ○ Caused by bacterial overgrowth and toxin production; risk factors include recent use of ampicillin and clindamycin, use of proton pump inhibitors (PPIs), and recent hospitalization.

  ○ Symptoms include fever, abdominal pain, profuse watery stools that can become bloody, and, in severe cases, development of pseudomembranous colitis. Symptoms can begin 4 to 8 weeks after start of antibiotics.

  ○ Flexible sigmoidoscopy shows nodular, inflammatory ulcers or yellow-white mucosal plaques.

– Others: See Table 5.1.

■ Drug induced: Possible causes include alcohol, phenolphthalein, castor oil, magnesium-containing antacids, caffeine, herbal tea, and broad-spectrum antibiotics (Goroll & Mulley, 2014).

• Chronic diarrhea (Table 5.1)

TABLE 5.1 Causes of Acute Versus Chronic Diarrhea

Acute Diarrhea	Chronic Diarrhea
Acute gastroenteritis	Irritable bowel syndrome
- Viral (e.g., norovirus,* rotavirus)	Inflammatory bowel disease
- Bacterial (e.g., Salmonella,* *Clostridium perfringens*,* and Campylobacter,* *Escherichia coli*, *C. difficile*)	Diabetic enteropathy
	Food intolerances
	Medications (e.g., lactulose intolerance)
- Parasite (*Giardia lamblia* – leading parasitic cause of diarrhea; causes stools to be watery or greasy; mucus is present)	Celiac disease
	Dumping syndrome (status post weight loss surgery)
- Drug-induced/alcohol	

*Most common according to CDC (2015).
Adapted from Goroll and Mulley (2014).

MANAGEMENT

Correcting dehydration and preventing worsened hydration status is the top priority when treating the patient with diarrhea. Most cases are self-limiting, and if patients are able to keep up with fluid losses, then further complications usually do not develop. Oral rehydration solutions are recommended to replace fluid losses and should include sugar, salt, and water (Wanke, 2015).

One option is 8 ounces of fruit juice with a pinch of salt, half a teaspoon of honey, or a teaspoon of table sugar. Another option is 8 ounces of water with a quarter teaspoon of baking soda (Goroll & Mulley, 2014).

There are some over-the-counter replacement solutions available, including Rehydralyte or Pedialyte (Wanke, 2015). Patients are instructed to avoid milk and dairy products for another 7 to 10 days after diarrhea has resolved, as there may be a component of lactose intolerance with acute diarrhea. Educate patient to eat high-carbohydrate foods like bananas, rice, baked potatoes, applesauce, and saltine crackers for a day or two prior to resuming a normal diet (Goroll & Mulley, 2014).

Antibiotics are rarely given for acute episodes of diarrhea. For management of traveler's diarrhea, however, Cipro 500 mg BID (twice a day) for 3 days or Bactrim DS BID for 3 days are options (Goroll & Mulley, 2014). Therapy for *C. difficile* is discontinuation of current antibiotics and starting either:

- Metronidazole 500 mg PO TID (per os three times a day) or 250 mg QID for (four times a day) 10 to 14 days for mild disease or
- Vancomycin 125 mg QID for 10 to 14 days for severe disease and/or recurrent episodes (Goroll & Mulley, 2014).

Probiotics have been shown to recolonize the intestine with healthy bacterial flora, which may have been lost from episodes of diarrhea (Wanke, 2015). There are several over-the-counter options available.

Multiple episodes of diarrhea cause perineal irritation and tenderness, even pain. It is important to teach patients the importance of perianal hygiene to provide comfort. Patients can use sitz baths after every bowel movement and as needed for discomfort.

Washing with a cloth or baby wipes instead of toilet paper can also provide some relief. Zinc oxide cream, hydrocortisone cream, and/or hemorroidal pads saturated with witch hazel can provide temporary pain relief in the perianal areas (Goroll & Mulley, 2014).

To slow down or reduce the frequency of diarrhea, loperamidine (Imodium) or atropine (Lomotil) can be used. These medications are not recommended if an inflammatory diarrheal illness is present as worsening of symptoms can occur (Han & Dubberke, 2013).

Admission to hospital may be necessary if the patient is unable to keep up with hydration, if postural hypotension is noted or develops, and there are signs of renal failure and bloody and/or purulent stools with fever. The very young and very old are most susceptible to severe complications of diarrhea (Goroll & Mulley, 2014).

ICD-10 CODE

Diarrhea, unspecified: R19.7
Enterocolitis due to *Clostridium difficile*: A04.7
Functional diarrhea: K59.1
Protozoal intestinal disease, unspecified: A07.9
Irritable bowel syndrome with diarrhea: K58.0
Irritable bowel syndrome without diarrhea: K58.9

═══════════════*FAST FACTS In a NUTSHELL*

1. Avoid dehydration as this is the most common reason for hospital admission in the patient with diarrhea.
2. Signs of inflammation and more serious illness are blood in the stool, fever, signs of hypovolemia, and severe abdominal pain.
3. Make helpful dietary recommendations, including suggestions for oral rehydration solutions and avoidance of dairy foods for a few days following illness.
4. Seek expert opinion when diarrhea persists for more than 4 weeks.

REFERENCES

Bonis, P. A., & Lamont, J. T. (2015). Approach to the adult with chronic diarrhea in developed countries. In S. Grover (Ed.) Waltham, MA: UpToDate. Retrieved from www.uptodate.com/contents/approach-to-the-adult-with-chronic-diarrhea-in-developed-countries?source=search_result&search=chronic+diarrhea&selectedTitle=1%7E150.html

Centers for Disease Control. (2015). Food safety homepage—Foodborne germs and illnesses. Retrieved from www.cdc.gov/foodsafety/foodborne-germs.html

Goroll, A. H., & Mulley, A. G. (2014). *Primary care medicine: Office evaluation and management of the adult patient* (7th ed., pp. 459–628). Philadelphia, PA: Lippincott Williams & Wilkins.

Gutierrez, R. L., Campbell, W. R., Cunningham, S. E., Riddle, M. S., & Young, P. E. (2015). Evaluation of acute infectious diarrhea. In P.R. McNally (Ed.), *GI/liver secrets plus* (5th ed., pp. 405–413). Philadelphia, PA: Elsevier Saunders.

Han, Z., & Dubberke, E. R. (2013). Infections of the gastrointestinal and hepatobiliary tract. In N. Kirmane, K. Woeltje, & H. Babcock (Eds.), *The Washington manual of infectious disease subspecialty consult* (pp. 109–140). Philadelphia, PA: Lippincott Williams & Wilkins.

Wanke, C. A. (2015). Approach to the adult with acute diarrhea in resource-rich countries. Retrieved from www.uptodate.com/contents/approach-to-the-adult-with-acute-diarrhea-in-resource-rich-countries?source=search_result&search=Approach+to+the+adult+with+acute+diarrhea&selectedTitle=1%7E150.html

Common GI Disorders

6

Celiac Disease

According to the American Gastroenterological Association (AGA), celiac disease is an intolerance to gluten that causes inflammation of the small bowel that can create malabsorption and poor digestion (AGA, 2006). Wheat, barley, and rye have gluten-containing products. Celiac disease is considered an autoimmune disorder with a genetic component. It is quickly becoming a common disorder that is gaining public recognition.

The food industry is taking notice, and there are many offerings now for gluten-free foods.

At the end of this chapter, the reader will be able to:

1. Name the gold standard laboratory test to diagnose celiac disease
2. State three risk factors for celiac disease
3. Describe the treatment for celiac disease

INCIDENCE AND RISK FACTORS

In the United States and worldwide, 1% of the population has celiac disease (AGA, 2006; Leffler & Vanga, 2015). There are several risk factors for the development of celiac disease

TABLE 6.1 Risk Factors for Celiac Disease

Cereal in infant's diet prior to 3 months of age	History of type 1 diabetes
First-degree relative with celiac disease	History of liver disease (elevated transaminases, primary biliary cirrhosis, autoimmune hepatitis)
History of iron-deficiency anemia	History of Down syndrome or Turner's syndrome
History of osteoporosis	History of autoimmune thyroid disease
History of other autoimmune disorders	History of fertility problems
Advanced age	North American or European ancestry
Immunoglobulin A deficiency	Eosinophilic esophagitis (children)

Adapted from AGA (2006), Leffler and Vanga (2015), and Schuppan et al. (2009).

(Table 6.1; AGA, 2006). If left untreated, patients with celiac disease have an increased risk of developing gastrointestinal cancers and enteropathy-associated T-cell lymphoma (Schuppan, Junker, & Barisani, 2009). In 40% to 50% of untreated patients with celiac disease, asymptomatic elevated aminotransferase levels develop (Leffler & Vanga, 2015).

ASSESSMENT FINDINGS

There is a wide range of symptoms for the patient with celiac disease. Some are asymptomatic, whereas some have severe malabsorption issues with skin manifestations. Celiac disease is frequently found in patients who have other autoimmune disorders (Schuppan et al., 2009).

Answers are needed regarding the patient's diet, paying particular attention to symptoms that develop following consumption of foods containing wheat, rye, or barley. Patients may complain of abdominal bloating, chronic or frequent episodes of diarrhea, and weight loss (Kelly, 2015).

Patients with severe gluten intolerance may develop a severely itchy rash (dermatitis herpetiformis; AGA, 2006).

Other issues include anemia, chronic fatigue, constipation, neurological/psychiatric issues (anxiety, migraines, peripheral neuropathy, ataxia), and infertility (Leffler & Vanga, 2015). All of these issues should be included in the review of systems when interviewing the patient with possible celiac disease.

On examination, providers evaluate for rash, abdominal distention, and evidence of weight loss (e.g., loose skin or temporal wasting; Kelly, 2015).

PERTINENT LABORATORY/DIAGNOSTIC FINDINGS

A serologic test called *immunoglobulin A* (IgA) *anti-tissue transglutaminase* (tTGA) is performed to detect possible celiac disease in patients over 2 years old (Kelly, 2015). The gold standard for diagnosing celiac disease is duodenal biopsy performed by endoscopy.

Characteristic histological changes of celiac disease are villous atrophy,* crypt hyperplasia, intraepithelial lymphocytosis, and mucosal inflammation. Biopsy is recommended in patients with a positive serologic test (AGA, 2006; Kelly, 2015; Schuppan et al., 2009).

DIFFERENTIAL DIAGNOSIS

Other possibilities for gastrointestinal symptoms that present with celiac disease include irritable bowel syndrome and lactose intolerance (Kelly, 2015).

MANAGEMENT

The only curative treatment for celiac disease is strict adherence to a gluten-free diet (GFD). As this disease has

*Villous atrophy is a hallmark finding in patients with celiac disease.

gained public awareness, there are many patient education pamphlets and even support groups available that patients can be a part of to help with diet adherence. It is important to recognize other vitamin deficiencies in patients with celiac disease, including B_{12}, D, iron, and folate. A screening for osteoporosis is also recommended by bone mineral density scan (AGA, 2006). Future treatments are being explored, including medications that could make it possible for these patients to tolerate gluten (Schuppan et al., 2009). Patients should consult with a registered dietician for a thorough dietary education on necessary lifestyle changes. With essential dietary changes, some patients may have undesired weight gain. Counseling on ideal food choices is important for patient success (Leffler & Vanga, 2015).

ICD-10 CODE

Celiac disease: K90.0

FAST FACTS in a NUTSHELL

1. Celiac disease is a common gastrointestinal disorder that results from gluten intolerance.
2. If left untreated, patients with celiac disease can develop cancer or have further serious complications.
3. The gold standard for diagnosing celiac disease is duodenal biopsy by endoscopy.
4. The only cure for celiac disease is strict adherence to a gluten-free diet.

REFERENCES

American Gastroenterological Association. (2006). AGA institute medical position statement on the diagnosis and management of celiac disease. *Gastroenterology, 131*, 1977–1980.

Kelly, C. P. (2015). Diagnosis of celiac disease in adults. In S. Grover (Ed.). Waltham, MA: UpToDate. Retrieved from www.uptodate.com /contents/diagnosis-of-celiac-disease-in-adults?source=search_ result&search=celiac&selectedTitle=1%7E150.html

Leffler, D. A., & Vanga, R. R. (2015). Celiac disease. In P. R. McNally (Ed.), *GI/liver secrets plus* (5th ed., pp. 308–312) McNally, P. R. (Ed.). Philadelphia, PA: Elsevier Saunders.

Schuppan, D., Junker, Y., & Barisani, D. (2009). Reviews in basic and clinical gastroenterology: Celiac disease: From pathogenesis to novel therapies. *Gastroenterology, 137*, 1912–1933.

7

Irritable Bowel Syndrome

Irritable bowel syndrome (IBS) is a common disorder. It is characterized as a functional disturbance of bowel motility with symptoms of lower abdominal pain and alternating episodes of diarrhea and constipation (Bonis & Lamont, 2015; Goroll & Mulley, 2014). Usually, patients with IBS have one predominant symptom, such as diarrhea, constipation, or abdominal pain. IBS is frequently associated with anxiety and somatization symptoms (Goroll & Mulley, 2014). It has been recommended that the diagnosis of IBS be considered in any patient who has "Abdominal pain or discomfort, Bloating, and Change in bowel habits" for the past six months (National Collaborating Centre for Nursing and Supportive Care, 2015, p. 7).

At the end of this chapter, the reader will be able to:

1. Define two guidelines used to diagnose IBS
2. Name two medication regimens that are FDA approved to treat IBS
3. Name a symptom that may be presented when evaluating the patient with IBS that is a red flag and requires consultation with an expert

INCIDENCE AND RISK FACTORS

IBS occurs in approximately 20% of the U.S. population (Goroll & Mulley, 2014). The onset of symptoms usually occurs in young adulthood, with females twice as likely as males to be diagnosed (Bonis & Lamont, 2015). IBS-C, or a chronic constipation disorder, affects 10% to 20% of the U.S. population. Risk factors for the development of IBS include alcohol consumption and high levels of psychological stress (Bonis & Lamont, 2015; Goroll & Mulley, 2014).

ASSESSMENT FINDINGS

Patients with IBS typically report bowel movements early in the morning or after a meal, and relate onset of symptoms with times of stress. Some patients report a sense of urgency prior to bowel movements and sometimes feel that emptying of stools was inadequate (Bonis & Lamont, 2015).

Diagnosis is made by history and physical examination. See Tables 7.1 and 7.2 for Manning criteria and Rome III criteria for IBS diagnosis. Physical examination may reveal abdominal distension and hyperactive bowel sounds (especially if patient is having an acute episode). Vital signs are usually normal. If fever is present, consider an inflammatory or infectious process.

TABLE 7.1 Manning Criteria

*More likely to be IBS when more criteria are met

Distension of the abdomen	Mucus-like stools
Pain relief after passage of stools	More frequent bowel movements when pain starts
Feeling of incomplete passage of stools	Looser bowel movements when pain starts

Source: Manning, Thompson, Heaton, and Morris (1978).

TABLE 7.2   Rome III Criteria for IBS Diagnosis

Patients meeting Rome III criteria must have had abdominal distress or pain at least 3 days per month for the past 3 months and meet at least two of the following conditions:
- Alternating diarrhea and constipation
- Pain or discomfort that improves after bowel movement
- Frequency of bowel movements is sporadic
- Beginning of symptoms related to change in frequency and/or stool characteristics
- Urgency with evacuation of stools
- Mucus-like stools
- Distension of abdomen

IBS, irritable bowel syndrome.
Adapted from Drossman (2006) and Longstreth et al. (2006).

PERTINENT LABORATORY/DIAGNOSTIC FINDINGS

If bloody stools are reported, then a complete blood count is necessary to rule out anemia. Also, if patient reports mucus-like or foul-smelling stools, electrolytes and other vitamin levels can be performed to evaluate for malabsorption issues. Other testing may include erythrocyte sedimentation rate (ESR), C-reactive protein (inflammatory markers), or celiac disease antibody markers (National Collaborating Centre for Nursing and Supportive Care, 2015). Esophagogastroduodenoscopy (EGD) and colonoscopy can be done to rule out other causes of diarrhea and/or constipation.

DIFFERENTIAL DIAGNOSIS

Patients report mucus-like stools with IBS. Patients who report bloody stools, greasy stools, or awaken in the middle of the night to have a bowel movement may have another disease process and not IBS. These types of symptoms are a red flag for inflammatory disease and may require expert consultation or urgent evaluation. Other red flags include unintentional weight loss, family history of ovarian or colon cancer, anemia, and abdominal or rectal masses noted on examination (National Collaborating Centre for Nursing and Supportive Care, 2015).

MANAGEMENT

The management of IBS depends mostly on symptom control, especially stress management. Dietary changes are necessary and include no alcohol or caffeine, avoidance of substances to which one is allergic, and an increase in dietary fiber intake. Patients should schedule regular meal times and should not skip meals. Adequate hydration is important. Some patients report relief from pain and abdominal distension with the use of probiotics. Patients with diarrhea issues should avoid artificial sweeteners (sorbitol). Biofeedback, behavioral techniques, and stress management are helpful in reducing the amount and severity of symptoms (Goroll & Mulley, 2014; National Collaborating Centre for Nursing and Supportive Care, 2015).

For IBS-D (diarrhea—predominant type), treatment options include loperamide and rifaximin (Goroll & Mulley, 2014). The American Gastroenterological Association (AGA) recommends rifaximin, alosetron, and loperamide as treatment options for these patients (Weinberg, Smalley, Heidelbaugh, & Sultan, 2014).

For IBS-C (predominant constipation), treatment options include linaclotide (Linzess), lubiprostone (Amitiza), osmotic laxatives, and biofeedback (Goroll & Mulley, 2014). The AGA recommends that these patients be treated with linaclotide or lubiprostone (Weinberg et al., 2014).

For any patient suffering from IBS, tricyclic antidepressants and antispasmodics can be tried to improve symptoms. The AGA does not recommend the use of selective serotonin reuptake inhibitors in patients with IBS (Weinberg et al., 2014). There is a high correlation of patients with IBS who also have psychiatric disorders, including depression, anxiety, and panic disorder (Padhy, Sahoo, Mahajan, & Sinha, 2015). Patients may need referral to a psychiatrist or psychologist to assist with symptom control.

EXPECTED OUTCOMES

Outcomes are expected to be good. Patients can have an optimal quality of life if symptoms are controlled.

ICD-10 CODE

Irritable bowel syndrome without diarrhea: K58.9
Irritable bowel syndrome with diarrhea: K58.0

================================= *FAST FACTS in a NUTSHELL*

1. Patients with IBS have a good prognosis and can live a normal life with symptom control and stress management.
2. There are several new U.S. Food and Drug Administration (FDA)-approved medications that are available to treat patients with IBS. Medication choice is dependent on the predominant symptom (diarrhea versus constipation).
3. Use of Rome III criteria and/or Manning criteria is helpful to determine whether IBS is a probable diagnosis in the patient with chronic diarrhea or constipation.

REFERENCES

Bonis, P. A., & Lamont, J. T. (2015). Approach to the adult with chronic diarrhea in developed countries. Retrieved from www.uptodate.com/contents/approach-to-the-adult-with-chronic-diarrhea-in-developed-countries?source=search_re

sult&search=Approach+to+the+adult+with+chronic&selectedTit
le=1%7E150.html

Drossman, D. A. (2006). The functional gastrointestinal disorders and the Rome III process. *Gastroenterology, 130*(5), 1377–1390.

Goroll, A. H., & Mulley, A. G. (2014). *Primary care medicine: Office evaluation and management of the adult patient* (7th ed., pp. 459–628). Philadelphia, PA: Lippincott Williams & Wilkins.

Longstreth, G. F., Thompson, W. G., Chey, W. D., Houghton, L. A., Mearin, F., & Spiller, R. C. (2006). Functional bowel disorders. *Gastroenterology, 130*(5), 1480–1491.

Manning, A. P., Thompson, W. G., Heaton, K. W., & Morris, A. F. (1978). Towards positive diagnosis of the irritable bowel. *British Medical Journal, 2*(6138), 653–654.

National Collaborating Centre for Nursing and Supportive Care. (2015). *Irritable bowel syndrome in adults: Diagnosis and management of irritable bowel syndrome in primary care.* London, England: National Institute for Health and Care Excellence (NICE).

Padhy, S. K., Sahoo, S., Mahajan, S., & Sinha, S. K. (2015). Irritable bowel syndrome: Is it "irritable brain" or "irritable bowel"? *Journal of Neurosciences in Rural Practice, 6*, 568–577.

Weinberg, D. S., Smalley, W., Heidelbaugh, J. J., & Sultan, S. (2014). American Gastroenterological Association Institute guideline on the pharmacological management of irritable bowel syndrome. *Gastroenterology, 147*, 1146–1148.

8

Food Intolerances
or Allergies

Food intolerances, or food allergies, are becoming increasingly common and recognized more frequently as a cause of gastrointestinal distress. Both immunological and nonimmunological reactions to food exist, with nonimmunological reactions occurring much more often. Reactions usually occur as the body's response to a food protein (Burks, 2015).

Nonimmunological reactions to food typically occur in the skin and gastrointestinal tract, and are usually not as severe.

Food intolerance is defined as an adverse reaction to a specific food. Celiac disease (see Chapter 6) and lactose intolerance are examples of food intolerances and are the most commonly diagnosed food intolerances (Rindfleisch, 2012).

At the end of this chapter, the reader will be able to:

1. Identify the most common food allergen (causing an immune response)
2. Name two other differential diagnoses to consider in the patient with a possible food allergy
3. State two possible treatment options for the patient with food-induced anaphylaxis

INCIDENCE AND RISK FACTORS

Food-induced anaphylaxis, particularly in the pediatric population, has increased over the past 50 years. It has been estimated that over 125,000 emergency room visits per year in the United States are related to a food-related reaction or allergy. Most common reactions occur from peanuts and tree nuts, followed by fish and shellfish allergies. Patients at risk are those who have asthma and/or a history of allergic reactions to food (Sampson, 2014). Food allergy reactions are increasing in our population, with 4% to 8% occurring in children and 1% to 4% occurring in adults (Rindfleisch, 2012).

ASSESSMENT FINDINGS

Symptoms can range from mild to severe anaphylactic-type reactions. Patients should be questioned regarding skin lesions, rash, difficulty breathing, palpitations, chest pain, nausea, vomiting, or diarrhea.

Patients with an immunological reaction to food develop symptoms acutely, usually within minutes to 2 hours after consumption of the offending food. Symptoms that may develop include an itchy rash (urticaria) and swelling (angioedema), asthma and allergic rhinitis, nausea, vomiting, abdominal pain and/or cramping, and diarrhea. The most severe reaction that can occur is an anaphylaxis reaction, which occurs quickly and can cause death if not treated rapidly (Burks, 2015).

PERTINENT LABORATORY FINDINGS

Immunologic testing—allergic reaction: enzyme-linked immunosorbent assay testing performed to determine presence of IgG and IgE immunoglobulins (Rindfleisch, 2012).

Antigen leukocyte cellular antibody test (ALCAT)—measures body's response to food antigens (Rindfleisch, 2012).

These tests should be ordered by an allergy specialist who can review findings in detail with patient and determine best treatment.

DIFFERENTIAL DIAGNOSIS

Differential diagnosis in patients with food intolerances is largely dependent on the type of reaction that is occurring. Some considerations include:

- Lactose intolerance
- Anatomic abnormalities
- Neurologic disorders
- Gastroesophageal reflux disease (GERD)
- Infectious processes, gastroenteritis
- Pancreatic insufficiency
- Peptic ulcer disease (Burks, 2015)

MANAGEMENT

The key to managing the patient with a food intolerance or allergy is to identify the trigger. An accurate dietary history (preferably a food diary) is important in identifying the possible allergen. Expert consultation to a specially trained allergist is recommended for uncertain or moderate to severe cases to accurately identify the food culprit causing the patient to become ill. Once the allergen or trigger is identified, the patient must avoid the allergen to prevent future episodes. For those patients with severe reactions, providers should prescribe an epinephrine injection for emergencies and provide patient and family education on proper usage. Patients should be told when to seek urgent medical attention.

For patients with food intolerance, an elimination diet may be recommended. A careful history should be reviewed with the patient and a plan of which foods to eliminate can be recommended based on symptoms. These foods should be avoided for a few weeks. Individual foods can be reintroduced gradually and, if symptoms recur, those foods should be avoided (Rindfleisch, 2012).

ICD-10 Code

Food allergy: Z91.02
Lactose intolerance, unspecified: E73.9
Hereditary fructose intolerance: E74.12
Malabsorption due to intolerance (to protein, fat, starch, carbohydrate, or not classified elsewhere): K90.4

FAST FACTS in a NUTSHELL

1. A careful dietary history is important when trying to determine a food allergy or intolerance. A food diary can be used and may provide a clue as to the offending allergen.
2. For patients with a severe food allergy history, a medical-alert bracelet is recommended for daily wear in combination with constant access to epinephrine injection in case of food allergen exposure.
3. An elimination diet may be recommended to retrain the body to avoid the offending food and to rid the body of its exposure.
4. Consultation with an allergist is recommended for moderate to severe cases or if symptoms have been prolonged or reoccur.

REFERENCES

Burks, W. (2015). Clinical manifestations of food allergy: An overview. Retrieved from www.uptodate.com/contents/clinical-manifestations-of-food-allergy-an-overview?source=search_result&search=Clinical+manifestations+of+food+allergy&selectedTitle=1%7E150.html

Rindfleisch, J. A. (2012). Food intolerance and elimination diet. In D. Rakel (Ed.), *Integrative medicine* (3rd ed., pp. 776–788). Philadelphia, PA: Saunders.

Sampson, H. A. (2014). Food-induced anaphylaxis. Retrieved from www.uptodate.com/contents/food-induced-anaphylaxis?source=search_result&search=food+induced+anaphylaxis&selectedTitle=1%7E40.html

9

Inflammatory Bowel Disease

Inflammatory bowel disease (IBD) is a broad diagnosis that includes two major chronic diseases: ulcerative colitis (UC) and Crohn's disease (CD). These disorders have some similarities, but also some major differences that require different management (Peppercorn & Cheifetz, 2015).

UC is a chronic inflammatory bowel disorder affecting the colon. Patients affected have flares or intermittent relapses (Peppercorn & Cheifetz, 2015). Patients may have mild symptoms with mucus-like or bloody diarrhea to a severe presentation with more than 10 bowel movements per day, fever, severe cramps, severe blood loss requiring blood transfusions, and weight loss with malnutrition issues (Bonis & Lamont, 2015).

CD is also a chronic inflammatory bowel disorder, but may involve the entire gastrointestinal tract. Patients typically have symptoms that include diarrhea, abdominal pain, weight loss, and fever (Bonis & Lamont, 2015).

At the end of this chapter, the reader will be able to:

1. State the difference between UC and CD
2. Name two risk factors for the development of IBD
3. Discuss the goal of medical management for the patient with IBD

INCIDENCE AND RISK FACTORS

IBD is typically diagnosed in young adulthood (15–40 years of age). It has a familial component, with individuals of Jewish ancestry being more commonly affected (Goroll & Mulley, 2014). Smoking has been associated with a higher risk of developing CD. Certain food antigens, particularly processed, sugary, and fried foods, have been associated with the development of IBD (Peppercorn & Cheifetz, 2015). Other associated risk factors may include stress, geographic latitude, use of nonsteroidal anti-inflammatory drugs (NSAIDs), low vitamin D, and depression (Goroll & Mulley, 2014).

There are over 1.6 million people in the United States with IBD (Bailey & Glasgow, 2015). Incidence rates in North America are high compared to Asian or Middle Eastern countries (Peppercorn & Cheifetz, 2015).

ASSESSMENT FINDINGS

UC is an inflammatory disease of the mucosa of the colon and rectum. Typical symptoms include bowel movement urgency, tenesmus (e.g., recurrent inclination to eliminate bowels), and bloody diarrhea. In severe cases, fever, anorexia, and weight loss can develop (Goroll & Mulley, 2014).

CD is a chronic inflammatory disorder of the alimentary tract. It is associated with high levels of proinflammatory cytokines. Discontinuous distribution is a key diagnostic finding of CD; affected areas of the bowel are scattered. These areas can be perforated and develop strictures and fistulas; even abscesses can develop. Patients can develop symptoms, including diarrhea and abdominal pain, weight loss, fever, vomiting, perianal discomfort, and bleeding (Goroll & Mulley, 2014).

On physical examination, patients who present at the onset of symptoms typically have a normal examination. Patients may report weight loss and/or abdominal tenderness (Goroll & Mulley, 2014). Other signs include mouth ulcers, rash, episcleritis, fistula, bloody stools, and signs of anemia (Bonis & Lamont, 2015).

Patients are questioned regarding history of bowel movements, including frequency and characteristics of stools, timing of bowel movements, and associated symptoms (including bloody stools, fevers, joint pain, mouth ulcers, or eye redness). Weight loss, recent travel history, or new medications/change in diet should be noted (Bonis & Lamont, 2015).

PERTINENT LABORATORY/DIAGNOSTIC FINDINGS

Consider complete blood count (to evaluate for anemia if bloody stools are present), erythrocyte sedimentation rate, thyroid function tests, and tests for electrolytes, total protein, and albumin (evaluating for nutrition deficiencies). Endoscopic evaluation may be needed if patient presents with moderate to severe symptoms or if there are ongoing issues (Bonis & Lamont, 2015). Referral to a gastroenterologist specializing in IBD may be needed.

To confirm diagnosis, a flexible sigmoidoscopy is necessary in cases of UC and a colonoscopy is necessary in cases of CD (Goroll & Mulley, 2014).

DIFFERENTIAL DIAGNOSIS

IBD differential diagnosis includes, but is not limited to:

- Hyperthyroidism
- Malabsorption
- HIV infection
- Type 1 diabetes
- Celiac disease
- Bacterial overgrowth
- Bacterial or viral gastroenteritis
- Infectious colitis
- Irritable bowel syndrome

MANAGEMENT

The goal for treatment of IBD is to suppress the immune system and help heal the bowel. Initial treatment for patients with mild to moderate UC includes 5-aminosalicyclic acid compounds (i.e., mesalamine, olsalazine, sulfasalazine, and balsalazide).

Other options are thiopurines, cyclosporine, methotrexate, and tumor necrosis factor antagonists (Grevenitis, Thomas, & Lodhia, 2015). For patients with CD, medications, such as budesonide, azathioprine, and prednisone, may be required (Sandborn, 2014).

Patients should be monitored closely for complications of IBD, including intestinal fistula (occurs only in CD), short bowel syndrome, pouch complications (occurring after proctocolectomy), and deep vein thrombosis. Moderate to severe cases and individuals who have failed medical therapy may need colorectal surgery (Bailey & Glasgow, 2015).

Patients are educated about IBD disease process and importance of medication compliance; awareness of possible complications is important for patient well-being.

ICD-10 CODE

Crohn's disease, unspecified without complications: K50.90
Crohn's disease, unspecified with abscess: K50.914
Crohn's disease, unspecified with other complication: K50.918
Crohn's disease, unspecified with fistula: K50.913
Crohn's disease, unspecified with unspecified complications: K50.919
Crohn's disease, unspecified with rectal bleeding: K 50.911
Ulcerative colitis, unspecified without complications: K51.90
Other ulcerative colitis with other complications: K51.818
Ulcerative colitis, unspecified with abscess: K51.914
Ulcerative colitis, with fistula: K51.813
Other ulcerative colitis with rectal bleeding: K51.811

1. Patients with complaints of bloody stool and chronic diarrhea lasting longer than 4 weeks should be investigated thoroughly for possible diagnosis of IBD.
2. Patients with UC have an increased risk of colorectal cancer.
3. The goal of treatment is to reduce risk of flares or exacerbations and to reduce risk of severe complications.
4. Nutrition modifications may need to be made for the patient with IBD. Patient education is important for well-being.

REFERENCES

Bailey, E. H., & Glasgow, S. C. (2015). Challenges in the medical and surgical management of chronic inflammatory bowel disease. *Surgical Clinics of North America, 95*, 1233–1244.

Bonis, P. A., & Lamont, J. T. (2015). Approach to the adult with chronic diarrhea in developed countries. Retrieved from www.uptodate.com/contents/approach-to-the-adult-with-chronic-diarrhea-in-developed-countries?source=search_result&search=Approach+to+the+adult+with+chronic&selectedTitle=1%7E150.html

Goroll, A. H., & Mulley, A. G. (2014). *Primary care medicine: Office evaluation and management of the adult patient* (7th ed., pp. 459–628). Philadelphia, PA: Lippincott Williams & Wilkins.

Grevenitis, P., Thomas, A., & Lodhia, N. (2015). Medical therapy for inflammatory bowel disease. *Surgical Clinics of North America, 95*, 1159–1182.

Peppercorn, M. A., & Cheifetz, A. S. (2015). Definition, epidemiology, and risk factors in inflammatory bowel disease. Retrieved from www.uptodate.com/contents/definition-epidemiology-and-risk-factors-in-inflammatory-bowel-disease?source=search_result&search=Definition%2C+epidemiology%2C+and+risk+factors+in+inflammatory&selectedTitle=1%7E150.html

Sandborn, W. J. (2014). Crohn disease evaluation and treatment: Clinical decision tool. *Gastroenterology, 147*(3), 702–705.

10

Gastroesophageal Reflux Disease

Gastroesophageal reflux disease (GERD) is a common condition in which stomach contents flow upward causing bothersome symptoms, including a burning sensation in the esophagus and throat, and other complications. Normally, the lower esophageal sphincter (LES) maintains a pressure barrier between the stomach and the esophagus. In GERD, several factors contribute to the symptoms: a reduction in resting LES tone, an inappropriate relaxation of LES, irritation caused by stomach acid, decreased peristalsis, and the gastrointestinal (GI) tract mucosa not being resistant to acids (Goroll & Mulley, 2014). Complications of GERD include Barrett's esophagus, peptic stricture, asthma, chronic cough, and esophageal adenocarcinoma (Niaz et al., 2015).

At the end of this chapter, the reader will be able to:

1. Define *GERD*
2. Evaluate treatment options for the patient with GERD
3. Name two potential complications of the patient with GERD

INCIDENCE AND RISK FACTORS

GERD is one of the most common conditions seen in primary care, affecting 10% to 20% of people in the United States (Harnik, 2015).

Risk factors include:

- Obesity
- Tobacco use
- Ethanol use
- Eating chocolate
- Ingesting high concentrations of fat or carbohydrates
- Eating citrus fruits (Goroll & Mulley, 2014)

ASSESSMENT

Patients with GERD often complain of heartburn, dysphagia (difficulty swallowing), and regurgitation. Other symptoms may include chest pain, nausea, excessive salivation, or the feeling of a lump in the throat. A thorough history and physical examination are essential for proper diagnosis and treatment. Diagnosis of GERD is made by clinical symptoms (Kahrilas, 2015).

IMAGING STUDIES

Upper endoscopy is warranted if the following conditions are present:

- Heartburn alarm symptoms (dysphagia, bleeding, anemia, weight loss, recurrent vomiting)
- Persistent GERD symptoms despite 4 to 8 weeks receiving a proton pump inhibitor (PPI) twice a day
- Severe erosive gastritis after 2 months' course of PPI—check for healing and check for Barrett's esophagus
- History of esophageal stricture with recurrent dysphagia (Goroll & Mulley, 2014)

Upper endoscopy results of the patient with GERD may show a normal examination, or signs of esophagitis, or even ulcers or erosions in the esophagus (Kahrilas, 2015).

DIFFERENTIAL DIAGNOSIS

The differential diagnosis of the patient with GERD may include infectious or eosinophilic esophagitis, cancer, peptic ulcer disease, coronary artery disease, or stricture motor impairment of the esophagus (Harnik, 2015; Kahrilas, 2015).

MANAGEMENT

Management of GERD includes several lifestyle modifications, including avoidance of foods thought to trigger symptoms (fatty or spicy foods, alcohol, chocolate, coffee, carbonated drinks, citrus fruits), weight reduction, smoking cessation, avoidance of large meals prior to bed, and elevating the head of the bed when lying down (American Gastroenterological Association, 2008; Goroll & Mulley, 2014). For medication management, most providers recommend prescribing a PPI twice a day for symptom control (American Gastroenterological Association, 2008). Antacids and H-2 receptor blockers are also options for more immediate symptom relief (Goroll & Mulley, 2014). Patients may need to be on therapy indefinitely to prevent complications (Harnik, 2015).

Antireflux surgery is an option for patients with GERD who are unable to take medications to treat the symptoms (American Gastroenterological Association, 2008; Goroll & Mulley, 2014).

Referral to a gastroenterologist is recommended for patients with suspected GERD whose symptoms do not respond to PPI therapy, patients with atypical symptoms, or symptoms such as weight loss, anemia of unknown etiology, hematemesis, difficulty swallowing, or epigastric mass (Harnik, 2015).

ICD-10 CODE

Gastroesophageal reflux disease without esophagitis: K21.9
Gastroesophageal reflux disease with esophagitis: K21.0

FAST FACTS in a NUTSHELL

1. GERD diagnosis is made by clinical presentation.
2. Many patients will need indefinite medical treatment with a PPI to prevent complications of GERD.
3. Providers should be aware of when referral to a specialist is required for further evaluation and treatment.

REFERENCES

American Gastroenterological Association. (2008). American Gastroenterological Association Institute technical review on the management of gastroesophageal reflux disease. *Gastroenterology, 135*, 1392–1413.

Goroll, A. H., & Mulley, A. G. (2014). *Primary care medicine: Office evaluation and management of the adult patient* (7th ed., pp. 459–628). Philadelphia, PA: Lippincott Williams & Wilkins.

Harnik, I. G. (2015). In the clinic: Gastroesophageal reflux disease. *Annals of Internal Medicine, 163*(1), ITC1. doi: 10.7326/AITC201507070

Kahrilas, P. J. (2015). Clinical manifestations and diagnosis of gastroesophageal reflux in adults. Retrieved from www.uptodate.com/contents/clinical-manifestations-and-diagnosis-of-gastroesophageal-reflux-in-adults?source=search_result&search=Clinical+manifestations+and+diagnosis+of+gastroesophageal&selectedTitle=2%7E150.html

Niaz, S. K., Quraishy, M. S., Taj, M. A., Abid, S., Alam, A., Nawaz, A. A., . . . Pakistan Society of Gastroenterology (GERD Consensus Group). (2015). Guidelines on gastroesophageal disease. *Journal of Pakistan Medical Association, 65*(5), 532–541.

Peptic Ulcer Disease

Peptic ulcer disease is a disorder of the gastric or duodenal mucosa in which alteration in the secretion of mucus, production of bicarbonate, and impaired cellular repair occurs. Some drugs, such as aspirin and nonsteroidal anti-inflammatory drugs (NSAIDs), have been blamed for peptic ulcer formation. Helicobacter pylori, *a bacteria, is capable of surviving in the gastric acid environment, and its presence in the gastrointestinal (GI) tract causes an inflammatory response resulting in apoptosis, or cellular death. Its presence has been associated with peptic ulcer formation (Goroll & Mulley, 2014). There are several serious complications of peptic ulcer disease that can develop if left untreated (Fashner & Gitu, 2015).*

At the end of the chapter, the reader will be able to:

1. Name two areas where peptic ulcers form
2. State a goal of treatment for patients with peptic ulcer disease
3. Name two options for medical management in the patient with peptic ulcer disease

INCIDENCE AND RISK FACTORS

With increased recognition and treatment of peptic ulcer disease and *H. pylori*, the prevalence of this disease has decreased in recent years. Peptic ulcer disease affects 2% of Americans, with males twice as likely to be affected as females, with a peak age of onset at 45 to 54 years. The most common peptic ulcers are duodenal ulcers (Goroll & Mulley, 2014).

Risk factors for the development of peptic ulcer disease are chronic NSAID use, older age, *H. pylori* infection, use of anticoagulant or antiplatelet medications, history of prior ulcers, use of corticosteroids, alcohol use, and smoking (Fashner & Gitu, 2015; Goroll & Mulley, 2014). Peptic ulcer disease is not caused by stress, emotional distress, or spicy foods (American College of Gastroenterology [ACG], 2016).

Complications that can develop if peptic ulcer disease is left untreated include gastrointestinal bleeding, gastric perforation, gastric cancer (untreated *H. pylori* infection), and gastric outlet obstruction, with bleeding the most common (Fashner & Gitu, 2015).

ASSESSMENT FINDINGS

Most patients with peptic ulcer disease are asymptomatic. When symptoms do arise, dyspepsia is a common complaint. Patients report feelings of burning, abdominal pain, epigastric pain relieved by antacids, and tenderness in the epigastric area. If *H. pylori* is suspected testing is recommended by the American College of Gastroenterology (ACG, 2016; Fashner & Gitu, 2015; Goroll & Mulley, 2014). Patients indicate that the pain occurs in clusters, with frequent pain-free periods. Duodenal ulcers typically cause pain that is relieved by food, but then the pain recurs 2 to 3 hours after a meal. Gastric ulcers typically cause pain during meals and the pain can radiate to epigastric and substernal areas. Pain is described as dull, gnawing, or burning. Patients may also complain of heartburn (Goroll & Mulley, 2014).

Physical examination may be normal, or patients may have epigastric tenderness with palpation. Noting epigastric mass, signs of anemia, or abnormal vital signs would be indications of a more serious problem that requires urgent medical care.

PERTINENT LABORATORY/DIAGNOSTIC FINDINGS

There are several tests available to determine the presence of *H. pylori*. The most common is the urea breath test, which is costly and inconvenient for some patients, as patients must fast for 6 hours prior to the test and not take proton pump inhibitor (PPI) medication for 2 weeks before the test. It is, however, commonly used on initial diagnosis and to ensure a cure following treatment. Another is serologic immunoglobulin G specific for *H. pylori*. Limitations of this test are that it cannot determine a new versus old infection. Referral to a gastroenterologist and an endoscopy with biopsies are recommended if the patient is older than 55 years, or if there are alarm symptoms (including difficulty or painful swallowing, weight loss, hematemesia, anemia of unknown etiology, or chest pain; Fashner & Gitu, 2015). Fecal occult blood testing and iron studies may be needed if anemic (Goroll & Mulley, 2014).

DIFFERENTIAL DIAGNOSIS

Differential diagnosis includes gastritis, esophagitis, functional dyspepsia, gastroenteritis, gastroesophageal reflux disease (GERD), celiac disease, irritable bowel syndrome, inflammatory bowel disease, perforation of the esophagus, cholangitis, gallstones, Barrett esophagus, gastric cancer, abdominal aortic aneurysm, acute coronary syndrome, and viral hepatitis (Fashner & Gitu, 2015).

MANAGEMENT

Lifestyle Modifications

Initial management is aimed at lifestyle changes, including eliminating use of aspirin and/or NSAIDs, alcohol, smoking cessation, reducing stress, and making dietary changes (avoid eating prior to bedtime, eat a bland diet, avoid spicy/acidic foods and beverages or other foods that cause pain and encourage small, frequent meals throughout the day; Goroll & Mulley, 2014). There is no definite diet recommended for patients with peptic ulcer disease (ACG, 2016).

Medications

One of the goals of treatment for the patient with peptic ulcer disease is eradication of *H. pylori* infection. There is a high resistance of *H. pylori* to metronidazole and clarithromycin, so recent changes have been made to recommended therapy (Goroll & Mulley, 2014). Standard triple therapy, including a PPI with two antibiotics for 7 to 10 days is first-line treatment for patients with a new diagnosis of peptic ulcer disease with known *H. pylori* infection. Patients are told to reduce the dose or stop taking NSAID medications (Table 11.1; Fashner & Gitu, 2015).

PPIs should be taken 30 minutes to an hour prior to a meal for optimal effectiveness. These medications are used to reduce acid production and stimulate tissue healing. Options are esomeprazole (Nexium), omeprazole (Prilosec), and pantoprazole (Protonix). Again drug-to-drug interactions are possible, so a careful review of all medications is necessary. Some studies have shown an association with long-term PPI use and infections,

---

TABLE 11.1 Treatment Options for *Helicobacter pylori* Eradication

- Option 1: Triple therapy: PPI BID for 7–14 days, amoxicillin 1 g BID for 7–14 days, and clarithromycin 500 mg BID for 7–14 days
- Option 2: Quadruple therapy: PPI BID for 10–14 days, tripotassiumdicitratobismuthate 120 mg QID 10–14 days, tetracycline 500 mg QID for 10–14 days, and metronidazole 250 mg QID 10–14 days
- Option 3: Sequential therapy

Days 1–5: PPI BID, amoxicillin 1 gm BID
Days 6–10: PPI BID, clarithromycin 500 mg BID, tinidazole 500 mg BID

PPI, proton pump inhibitor; BID, twice a day; QID, four times a day.

Adapted from Fashner and Gitu (2015) and Goroll and Mulley (2014).

including *Clostridium difficile* and community-acquired pneumonia (Goroll & Mulley, 2014).

Histamine-2 blockers (e.g., cimetidine, ranitidine, and famotidine) are medications to reduce acid production and may be prescribed in certain cases, especially if the patient has a duodenal ulcer (ACG, 2016). These medications are known to cause drug-to-drug interactions, so a review of all medications is necessary prior to prescribing. Antacids can be used as well. Timing is important with these medications. For optimal effectiveness, give 1 hour after eating and/or 3 hours after a meal. Some side effects include diarrhea and phosphate depletion (Goroll & Mulley, 2014).

Sucralfate, a formula of aluminum hydroxide and sulfated sucrose, has been given to patients with peptic ulcer disease to protect the gastric and duodenal mucosa. A common side effect is constipation.

Expected Outcomes

When *H. pylori* is present, there is an additional risk for development of antral gastritis, which is a risk factor for gastric cancer and mucosa-associated lymphoid tissue lymphoma. After *H. pylori* is treated, most patients recover well. If treatment is not working or if there are alarm signs, referral to a GI specialist is recommended.

Admission to the hospital may be necessary if there are complications such as GI bleeding (vomiting blood or black emesis, black tarry stools), hypotension, tachycardia (signs of anemia), or signs of peritoneal irritation or gastric outlet obstruction. Consultation with a surgeon and gastroenterologist may be indicated (Goroll & Mulley, 2014).

ICD-10 CODE

Personal history of peptic ulcer disease: Z87.11
Acute peptic ulcer, with hemorrhage: K27.0
Chronic or unspecified peptic ulcer, with hemorrhage: K27.4
Acute peptic ulcer, site unspecified with perforation: K27.1

Chronic or unspecified peptic ulcer, with perforation: K27.5

Acute peptic ulcer, without hemorrhage or perforation: K27.3

Chronic or unspecified peptic ulcer, without hemorrhage or perforation: K27.7

Peptic ulcer, site unspecified, unspecified as acute or chronic, without perforation or hemorrhage: K27.9

Acute peptic ulcer, site unspecified, with both hemorrhage and perforation: K27.2

Chronic peptic ulcer, site unspecified, with both hemorrhage and perforation: K27.6

Helicobacter pylori as the cause of diseases classified elsewhere: B96.81

FAST FACTS in a NUTSHELL

1. Diagnosis of peptic ulcer disease is usually by history and physical examination.
2. Providers must be aware of alarm symptoms to effectively triage patients.
3. *H. pylori* must be eradicated to ensure patient improvement and to prevent complications.
4. A careful medication review is important for all patients, but particularly the elderly who are on several medications and who have been taking NSAIDs chronically.

REFERENCES

American College of Gastroenterology. (2016). Peptic ulcer disease. Retrieved from http://patients.gi.org/topics/peptic-ulcer-disease.html

Fashner, J., & Gitu, A. C. (2015). Diagnosis and treatment of peptic ulcer disease and *H. pylori* infection. *American Family Physician, 91*(4), 236–242.

Goroll, A. H., & Mulley, A. G. (2014). *Primary care medicine: Office evaluation and management of the adult patient* (7th ed., pp. 459–628). Philadelphia, PA: Lippincott Williams & Wilkins.

12

Diverticular Disease

Diverticulosis *is defined as the presence of diverticula (or outpouching areas in the colon). Occasional issues may include abdominal pain and/or constipation.* Diverticulitis *is defined as inflammation and infection of the diverticula (Goroll & Mulley, 2014). Acute diverticulitis presents as new-onset left lower quadrant pain, tenderness, fever, and leukocytosis. There may be additional inflammatory markers that are elevated (e.g., C-reactive protein [CRP]; Collins & Winter, 2015; Goroll & Mulley, 2014).*

At the end of this chapter, you will be able to:

1. State the difference between diverticulosis and diverticulitis
2. Name two assessment findings of the patient with diverticulitis
3. Describe the treatment for acute diverticulitis

INCIDENCE AND RISK FACTORS

Worldwide, it appears that diverticular disease is increasing. It is the third most common gastrointestinal (GI) disorder necessitating hospitalization, resulting in a large economic burden. Males are more likely than females to develop this disease and at a younger age (Collins & Winter, 2015).

The average age of an acute episode of diverticulitis is 63 (Pemberton & Young-Fadok, 2015).

There is a higher association of complications with diverticular disease in patients who smoke. Patients with irritable bowel syndrome (IBS) and irritable bowel disease (IBD) have a higher likelihood of having diverticular disease. Other risk factors include genetics, ethnicity, obesity, lack of physical activity, alcohol intake, and use of aspirin or nonsteroidal anti-inflammatory drugs (NSAIDs; Collins & Winter, 2015).

ASSESSMENT FINDINGS

The most common symptom for a patient with acute diverticulitis is abdominal pain, usually to the left lower quadrant. Other symptoms may include low-grade fever, nausea, vomiting, change in bowel (constipation or diarrhea), or urinary symptoms (dysuria, urgency, or frequency; Pemberton & Young-Fadok, 2015).

PERTINENT LABORATORY/DIAGNOSTIC FINDINGS

Diverticular disease diagnosis is made by history and physical examination (Goroll & Mulley, 2014).

Initially, ultrasound and CT scan are useful studies to determine degree of diverticulitis and whether there have been complications, including bowel obstruction, perforation, or abscess formation (Collins & Winter, 2015).

Colonoscopy has been recommended for patients 6 to 8 weeks after an acute diverticulitis episode to ensure there is no malignancy and to confirm diagnosis (Collins & Winter, 2015).

Laboratory testing includes complete blood count, electrolytes, and urinalysis. For women of childbearing age, a pregnancy test is completed (Pemberton & Young-Fadok, 2015).

Differential diagnosis for diverticular disease includes acute appendicitis, IBD, colitis (ischemic or infectious), ectopic pregnancy, colorectal cancer, or nephrolithiasis (Pemberton & Young-Fadok, 2015).

MANAGEMENT

For patients with diverticulosis, experts recommend increasing fiber intake, regular exercise, and avoidance of laxatives or enemas. Patients are taught to report fever, tenderness, or bleeding issues (Goroll & Mulley, 2014).

For patients with diverticulitis, experts recommend a clear-liquid diet initially and an antibiotic regimen (Table 12.1). There have been recent reports that antibiotics should be used selectively, rather than for every patient with a diagnosis of diverticulitis. A high-fiber diet as well as increasing physical activity are recommended to avoid further complications. Patients should avoid eating nuts, seeds, or popcorn as well as avoid use of NSAIDs (Stollman, Smalley, Hirano, & AGA Institute Clinical Guidelines Committee, 2015).

Patients with a temperature greater than 101°F, worsening abdominal pain, and/or signs of peritoneal irritation/inflammation should be hospitalized. If patients have leukocytosis, a CT scan should be obtained and urgent consultation with a surgeon arranged.

TABLE 12.1 Antibiotics for Diverticulitis
Broad-spectrum antibiotics for diverticulitis
• Bactrim 160/800 BID or Cipro 500 mg BID + Flagyl 500 mg QID × 7–10 days OR • Amoxicillin/clavulanate 875/125 mg BID for 7–10 days
BID, twice a day; QID, four times a day.

EXPECTED OUTCOMES

Patients with diverticular disease have a good prognosis. Over 70% of patients respond well to conservative treatment (Pemberton & Young-Fadok, 2015).

Hospital admission is necessary if there is lower GI bleeding, temperature greater than 101°F on oral antibiotic therapy, is unable to take fluids orally, has worsening abdominal pain, and peritoneal signs are present (Goroll & Mulley, 2014).

ICD-10 CODE

Diverticulosis of large intestine without perforation or abscess: K57.30

Diverticulosis of intestine, part unspecified, without perforation or abscess: K57.90

Diverticulosis of small intestine, without perforation or abscess: K57.10

Diverticulosis of both small and large intestine without perforation or abscess: K57.50

Diverticulitis of intestine, part unspecified, with perforation and abscess with bleeding: K57.81

Diverticulitis of small intestine with perforation and abscess with bleeding: K57.01

Diverticulitis of large intestine with perforation and abscess with bleeding: K57.21

Diverticulitis of intestine, part unspecified, without perforation or abscess: K57.92

Diverticulitis of both small and large intestine, without perforation or abscess with bleeding: K57.53

FAST FACTS in a NUTSHELL

1. In acute diverticulitis, abdominal pain is the most common complaint.
2. To confirm a diagnosis of acute diverticulitis, abdominal imaging is required.
3. Patients who have had diverticulitis should make lifestyle changes to prevent further episodes and to reduce the risk of complications.

REFERENCES

Collins, D., & Winter, D. C. (2015). Modern concepts in diverticular disease. *Journal of Clinical Gastroenterology, 49*(5), 358–369.

Goroll, A. H., & Mulley, A. G. (2014). *Primary care medicine: Office evaluation and management of the adult patient* (7th ed., pp. 459–628). Philadelphia, PA: Lippincott Williams & Wilkins.

Pemberton, J. H., & Young-Fadok, T. (2015). Clinical manifestations and diagnosis of acute diverticulitis in adults. Retrieved from www.uptodate.com/contents/clinical-manifestations-and-diagnosis-of-acute-diverticulitis-in-adults?source=search_result&search=diverticulitis&selectedTitle=3%7E42.html

Stollman, N., Smalley W., Hirano, I., & AGA Institute Clinical Guidelines Committee. (2015). American Gastroenterological Association Institute guideline on the management of acute diverticulitis. *Gastroenterology, 149*(7), 1944–1949.

13

Gallstones

Gallstones are very common in the United States. When discussing gallstone disease, there are several issues that can arise. The presence of gallstones is called choleli-thiasis, which is usually found incidentally on imaging studies. Conditions that require more urgent evaluation include biliary colic (pain associated with gallstones in the gallbladder), acute cholecystitis (inflammation of the gallbladder), choledocholithaisis (gallstones in the com-mon bile duct), cholangitis, and gallstone pancreatitis.

At the end of this chapter, you will be able to:

1. State the difference between cholelithiasis and cholecystitis
2. Describe when a cholecystectomy is surgically indicated
3. Name two lifestyle modifications that are recommended in the patient with gallstones

INCIDENCE AND RISK FACTORS

Cholelithiasis, or the presence of gallstones in the gallbladder, occurs in over 20 million Americans. In the United States, 500,000 patients have a cholecystectomy each year. The three Fs known to be associated with gallstones are fat, forty, and female. Those most commonly affected are obese middle-aged women (Goroll & Mulley, 2014). Individuals who are Native American, Hispanic, or Caucasian are most affected. Other risk factors include age (individuals older than 40 years), being female, pregnancy, sedentary lifestyle, use of oral contraceptives or estrogen replacement therapy, family history of gallstones, diabetes, cirrhosis, Crohn's disease, obesity, individuals who have a rapid weight loss (bariatric surgery), parenteral nutrition, and medications such as clofibrate, ceftriaxone, and octreotide (Afdhal, 2015; Goroll & Mulley, 2014).

ASSESSMENT FINDINGS

Patients usually are asymptomatic. However, when symptoms do occur, epigastric and/or right upper quadrant abdominal pain that is rapid in onset (called biliary colic) occurs and is associated with nausea and vomiting. It is important for the provider to be aware of the difference between biliary colic and complicated gallbladder disease. If abdominal pain lasts longer than 4 to 6 hours and/or is associated with a fever, urgent evaluation is needed (referral to the emergency room). Progression of symptoms could mean the onset of acute cholecystitis (Goroll & Mulley, 2014).

Choledocholithaisis, or gallstone in the common bile duct, causes abdominal pain as mentioned, but is also associated with elevated liver function tests and bilirubin levels (Goroll & Mulley, 2014). If left untreated, biliary fluid could back up causing biliary sludge and cholangitis. Cholangitis then can progress to bacteremia and sepsis.

Although some patients are asymptomatic, many patients with gallbladder disease have right upper quadrant abdominal pain, nausea, and vomiting. History is obtained with questions aimed at investigating the onset and duration of pain, as well as aggravating and alleviating factors. Associated symptoms are noted, including fever, nausea, vomiting, yellowing of skin or eyes, or itching (common with jaundice).

Physical examination findings of the patient with gallbladder disease may be fairly benign. More urgent signs, however, include abnormal vital signs (fever, tachycardia, and hypotension could be signs of infection or sepsis), jaundice and icteric sclera (signs of common bile duct blockage or cholangitis), right upper quadrant pain/tenderness to palpation, abdominal guarding, or a positive Murphy's sign.

PERTINENT LABORATORY/DIAGNOSTIC FINDINGS

Initial laboratory testing in patients with gallbladder disease includes a complete blood count, comprehensive metabolic panel, amylase, and lipase. Further testing may be needed if abnormal studies are present. In patients with suspected cholangitis, blood cultures are recommended to determine whether bacteremia is present.

An ultrasound scan is recommended for patients with suspected gallbladder disease. Further imaging may be required if abnormal results are found. Findings of acute cholecystitis include gallbladder wall thickening, pericholecystic fluid, and/or positive sonographic Murphy's sign. If there is concern about bile duct obstruction, a magnetic resonance cholangiopancreatography (MRCP) can be performed (Goroll & Mulley, 2014).

MANAGEMENT

Some factors protective against the development of gallstones have been discovered. These include vitamin C (ascorbic acid), eating nuts and vegetable proteins, coffee, and use of a statin (Afdhal, 2015). For the asymptomatic patient with cholelithiasis, lifestyle changes are recommended, including weight loss, avoidance of fatty foods, and smoking and alcohol cessation (Goroll & Mulley, 2014). Discontinuation of hormones (contraceptives or replacement therapy) is necessary.

For patients with biliary colic, surgery is usually not indicated unless symptoms are moderate to severe. Hospital admission is required for patients with acute cholecystitis, for administration of intravenous (IV) antibiotics and a surgical consultation. Usually a laparoscopic cholecystectomy is performed. In patients with choledocholithaisis, an endoscopic retrograde cholangiopancreatography (ERCP) is performed to remove the stone and debris from the common bile duct (UMHS Gallstone Guidelines, 2014).

ICD-10 CODE

Cholecystitis, unspecified: K81.9
Acute cholecystitis: K81.0
Chronic cholecystitis: K81.1
Other cholelithiasis with obstruction: K80.81
Other cholelithiasis without obstruction: K 80.80
Obstruction of bile duct: K83.1
Obstruction of gallbladder: K82.0
Biliary acute pancreatitis: K85.1

FAST FACTS in a NUTSHELL

1. *Cholelithiasis* refers to the presence of gallstones. Cholecystitis is the inflammation of the gallbladder.
2. If symptoms of biliary colic last longer than 4 to 5 hours and/or is associated with fever, urgent referral to the nearest emergency room is recommended.
3. Patients who have undergone bariatric surgery and/ or have had a rapid weight loss are at high risk for developing gallstone disease.
4. Lifestyle changes are important for all patients with gallstone disease, even after surgery.

REFERENCES

Afdhal, N. H. (2015). Epidemiology of and risk factors for gallstones. Retrieved from www.uptodate.com/contents/epidemiology-of-and-risk-factors-for-gallstones?source=search_result&search=Epidemiology+of+and+risk+factors+for+gallstones.&selectedTitle=1%7E150.html

Goroll, A. H., & Mulley, A. G. (2014). *Primary care medicine: Office evaluation and management of the adult patient* (7th ed., pp. 459–628). Philadelphia, PA: Lippincott Williams & Wilkins.

UMHS Gallstone Guideline. (2014). Evaluation and management of gallstone-related diseases in non-pregnant adults. Retrieved from www.med.umich.edu/1info/FHP/practiceguides/gallstone/Gallstonefinal.pdf

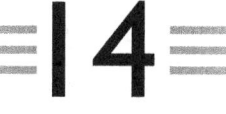

Gastrointestinal Cancers

The five most common gastrointestinal (GI) cancers are esophageal, gastric, pancreatic, colorectal, and hepatocellular carcinoma. Esophageal cancer has an association with chronic gastroesophageal reflux disease (GERD) and Barrett's esophagus. Gastric cancer is associated with untreated Helicobacter pylori *infection and consumption of high-salt foods. Pancreatic cancer is the fourth leading cause of cancer death in the United States. Most tumors are caused by the exocrine ductal epithelium as adenocarcinoma (Goroll & Mulley, 2014).*

Colorectal cancer is the third leading cause of cancer death in the United States and is associated with adenomatous polyps (Goroll & Mulley, 2014). Hepatocellular carcinoma is the fifth most common cancer and is described in detail in Chapter 28.

At the end of this chapter, the reader will be able to:

1. Name the most common GI cancer in the United States
2. State three risk factors for the development of colorectal cancer
3. Name the only GI cancer that has a screening test available

INCIDENCE AND RISK FACTORS

There are 14,000 new cases of esophageal cancer annually in the United States. Risk factors include Caucasian origin, male gender, older age, smoking, excessive alcohol consumption, and history of Barrett's esophagus (Goroll & Mulley, 2014).

There are 23,000 new cases of gastric cancer annually in the United States and 14,000 resultant deaths every year. Risk factors include chronic GERD, long-standing *H. pylori* infection, consumption of high-salt and salt-preserved foods, nitrate-cured or nitrate-processed meats, smoking, Epstein–Barr virus infection, Billroth II surgery, obesity, pernicious anemia (can lead to chronic atrophic gastritis), and familial adenomatous polyposis (Goroll & Mulley, 2014).

Pancreatic cancer is a devastating disease, with 45,000 new cases every year in the United States. There is a high mortality rate of 98%, usually because symptoms do not manifest until late in the disease process. Risk factors include genetic mutations—BRCA1 and 2, p16, MLH1, MSH2, PMS2; familial pancreatitis; Peutz–Jeghers syndrome; smoking; obesity; chronic exposure to dry-cleaning materials and gasoline-related compounds; and prior radiation exposure (Goroll & Mulley, 2014).

Colorectal cancer is the most common of the gastrointestinal cancers, with over 130,000 people being diagnosed each year. It is the second leading cause of cancer death among men and women in the United States. The median age of colorectal cancer diagnosis is 70. Americans have a 1:20 lifetime risk for developing colorectal cancer. Risk factors include a high-fat, low-fiber diet, obesity, tobacco use, heavy alcohol use, type 2 diabetes mellitus, advancing age, family history (first-degree relative increases risk twofold; increased risk if diagnosed before 60 years of age and increased further if younger than 50 years and if more than one relative), adenomatous polyps (precursor lesion), familial adenomatous polyposis (FAP) and Lynch syndrome, ulcerative colitis, Crohn's disease, and history of prior colorectal cancer (Goroll & Mulley, 2014).

Unfortunately, many times the patient with a gastrointestinal cancer is asymptomatic. There is no screening test for GI cancers except for colorectal cancer, making early diagnosis very difficult.

As always, a thorough history and physical examination are important. Patient report of bloody stool is a red flag of possible colorectal cancer. Complaints of severe abdominal pain or cramps, unintended weight loss, change in bowels with alternating constipation and diarrhea episodes, abdominal bloating, heartburn, persistent nausea with or without vomiting, lack of appetite, and ongoing weakness and fatigue are all potential symptoms of cancer and should not be ignored.

PERTINENT LABORATORY/DIAGNOSTIC FINDINGS

Routine laboratory data should be obtained as a baseline, including a complete blood count, comprehensive metabolic panel, and liver function testing.

There is no screening test available for esophageal cancer. It is recommended that for patients with a history of GERD longer than 5 years and for older White males with a history of smoking and excess alcohol use, an endoscopy with biopsy be performed. For those patients with Barrett's esophagus, a repeat esophagogastroduodenoscopy (EGD) is recommended every 3 months to 3 years depending on the degree of dysplagia.

For both gastric and pancreatic cancer, there is poor evidence on how and whom to screen for these diseases.

Colonoscopy is the gold standard screen for colorectal cancer. The U.S. Preventive Services Task Force (USPSTF) recommends colonoscopy every 10 years, starting at age 50 (45 years of age if African American) and a yearly fecal occult blood test (FOBT), with a potential for more frequent testing if polyps are found. If a patient has a positive occult blood test, a colonoscopy is recommended.

Educating patients on the need for colonoscopy is important. Some patients will avoid having this procedure because of time restraints (needing to take off work for test and need for a driver after procedure), embarrassment, and lack of resources or finances; even disparities among racial and socioeconomic groups may be present.

MANAGEMENT

All patients with GI cancers should have follow-up by an oncologist and a gastroenterology specialist. There is no screening tool available to screen for gastric, esophageal, or pancreatic cancers. In cases of pancreatic cancer, surgery is the only curative method; however, only 20% of patients are alive after 2 years. There are some studies that have associated a risk reduction of colorectal cancer and use of aspirin (Goroll & Mulley, 2014).

To reduce the risk of developing GI cancers, some lifestyle changes can be made. These include smoking cessation, eliminating alcohol, reducing fat intake, increasing fiber intake and consumption of fruits and vegetables, and exercising regularly (American Society for Gastrointestinal Endoscopy, 2014).

EXPECTED OUTCOMES

Unfortunately, many GI cancers are found late in the disease process and, as a result, patients have a poor prognosis. Less than 10% of patients with esophageal cancer survive after 5 years. Only 20% of patients with pancreatic cancer survive after 2 years. In patients with colorectal cancer, usually the cancer has spread beyond the intestinal wall when symptoms develop. At this stage, many patients will not survive past 5 years (Goroll & Mulley, 2014). This is why the screening tests are so important.

ICD-10 CODE

Malignant neoplasm of cardia: C16.0
Malignant neoplasm of esophagus: C15.9

Malignant neoplasm of body of stomach: C16.2
Malignant neoplasm of colon: C18.9
Malignant neoplasm of colon with rectum: C19
Malignant neoplasm of body of pancreas: C25.1
Malignant neoplasm of pancreas, unspecified: C25.9

===== *FAST FACTS in a NUTSHELL*

1. Lifestyle modifications are recommended to reduce the risk of developing GI cancers.
2. Colon polyps are precursors to colorectal cancer.
3. Colonoscopy is the gold standard for colorectal cancer screening.
4. Providers must take the time to educate patients on getting colonoscopies for colorectal screening.

REFERENCES

American Society for Gastrointestinal Endoscopy. (2014). Media backgrounder: Colorectal cancer screening. Retrieved from www.asge.org/press/press.aspx?id=552

Goroll, A. H., & Mulley, A. G. (2014). *Primary care medicine: Office evaluation and management of the adult patient* (7th ed., pp. 459–628). Philadelphia, PA: Lippincott Williams & Wilkins.

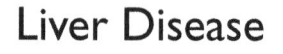

PART

III

Liver Disease

15

Assessment of Liver Function and Abnormal Liver Function Tests

The liver is located in the right upper quadrant of the abdomen and weighs approximately 2.5 to 3.5 pounds. It has several important functions, including the following:

- *Production and release of proteins (needed for proper clotting), vitamins, and enzymes*
- *Formation and release of bile (helps digestion of fat)*
- *Filtration and detoxification of medications and other substances in the body*
- *Construction and breakdown of cholesterol*
- *Creation and breakdown of lipids and glucose (metabolism of energy; gluconeogenesis; Sicklick, D'Angelica, & Fong, 2012)*

Liver function tests (LFTs) can be difficult to understand and apply clinically. The LFT is a combination of serum testing, including alkaline phosphate, alanine aminotransferase (ALT or serum glutamic pyruvic transaminase [SGPT]), aspartate aminotransferase (AST or serum glutamic oxaloacetic transaminase [SGOT]), and bilirubin levels (including total and direct). Other laboratory tests performed to evaluate liver function include prothrombin time (PT) and international normalized ratio (INR), gamma-glutamyltranspeptidase

(GGT), 5'-nucleotidase, albumin, and lactate dehydrogenase. Mild elevations in alkaline phosphate, ALT, and AST levels are seen commonly in primary care settings. With one abnormal reading, it is not necessary to refer patients to a specialist. Abnormal LFT results can occur for a variety of reasons. This chapter reviews liver testing and some reasons for these abnormalities.

At the end of this chapter, the reader will be able to:

1. Name the components of a liver profile
2. Identify two causes of an abnormal liver profile
3. State one reason for the patient with an abnormal liver profile to seek expert consultation

LIVER FUNCTION TESTS

Alkaline phosphatase (sometimes called *alk phos*) is a serum level that is derived from bone and liver cells. The normal range is 30 to 115 units/L. There are some elevations that result from placental secretion during pregnancy. In patients with blood type O or B, these levels can be increased following a fatty meal. Patients with diabetes can have mild elevations. In children and adolescents, alkaline phosphate can show mild elevations caused by rapid bone growth. Elevations can also be seen in patients who have biliary issues (American Gastroenterological Association, 2002; Fiellin, Reid, & O'Connor, 2000; Friedman, 2015; Pratt & Kaplan, 2000).

In patients who have acute liver injury, providers will see elevations of ALT and AST. ALT and AST are enzymes that are released from hepatocytes when injury occurs. Normal ranges for ALT are 10 to 50 units/L and 10 to 40 units/L for AST. Albumin is a protein that is produced by the liver. Low levels are seen in patients who have chronic liver disease, malnutrition, or cancer. Normal levels of albumin are

3.3 to 5.0 g/dL. Another important laboratory marker for liver injury is the INR. The normal INR range is 0.8 to 1.2. The liver normally produces protein that assists with proper blood clotting; when there is liver failure, these proteins are no longer formed and the patient's INR becomes dangerously high (American Gastroenterological Association, 2002; Fiellin, Reid, & O'Connor, 2000; Friedman, 2015; Pratt & Kaplan, 2000).

ASSESSMENT FINDINGS

In the patient with abnormal LFT results, providers should obtain a thorough history. Questions should include information on alcohol consumption, dietary recall (if there are signs of hepatitis A), social history (including sexual history if there is concern about viral hepatitis), history of blood transfusions, and medication history (including illicit drug use and over-the-counter and herbal medications; American Gastroenterological Association, 2002; Fiellin, Reid, & O'Connor, 2000; Friedman, 2015; Pratt & Kaplan, 2000).

Physical examination may be completely benign. If elevations of bilirubin levels are noted, patients may exhibit signs of jaundice (yellowing of skin, icteric sclera), and complain of intense itching (resulting from bile salt deposits in the tissue) American Gastroenterological Association, 2002; Fiellin, Reid, & O'Connor, 2000; Friedman, 2015; Pratt & Kaplan, 2000.

Why does the patient have abnormal LFTs? Further testing is done to try and answer this question. Viral hepatitis serology, complete blood count, prothrombin time (PT)/INR, albumin levels, iron studies, toxicology and alcohol screening, and autoimmune markers can be obtained. If history reveals that the patient just started a new medication (e.g., herbal medication, antibiotic, or statin), the patient should discontinue the medication and repeat blood work in 4 to 6 weeks (American Gastroenterological Association, 2002; Fiellin, Reid, & O'Connor, 2000; Friedman, 2015; Pratt & Kaplan, 2000).

IMAGING STUDIES

Imaging studies that are frequently ordered for the patient with abnormal LFT results are an initial abdominal ultrasound and/or CT scan if further imaging is required (American Gastroenterological Association, 2002; Fiellin, Reid, & O'Connor, 2000; Friedman, 2015; Pratt & Kaplan, 2000).

ABNORMAL LFT RESULTS

When abnormal LFT results are noted, providers must determine whether this is acute (less than 6 months) or chronic (longer than 6 months). Most patients are asymptomatic and have a benign physical examination. Usually, abnormal LFT results can be blamed on one of the following four factors:

- Disease
- Infection
- Drugs
- Pregnancy (American Gastroenterological Association, 2002; Fiellin, Reid, & O'Connor, 2000; Friedman, 2015; Pratt & Kaplan, 2000)

DIFFERENTIAL DIAGNOSIS

Mild elevations are seen in patients with chronic hepatitis B or C, fatty liver disease, or alcoholic cirrhosis. High elevations of ALT and AST (greater than 1,000) can be seen in patients with acute liver failure resulting from drugs, also called *shock liver*, acute hepatitis A or B, or ischemic liver injury. Patients with an elevated bilirubin level typically also have elevations of alkaline phosphatase. These elevations can be seen in patients with viral hepatitis and drug-related liver injury (herbal or alcohol). High elevations of bilirubin levels can be seen in patients with hepatocellular carcinoma; cholangiocarcinoma; viral hepatitis; pregnancy; those receiving total parenteral nutrition; and biliary diseases, including primary sclerosing cholangitis, primary biliary cirrhosis, or cholangitis. In patients with a high level of indirect or unconjugated bilirubin levels, there is typically an overproduction of bilirubin (hemolysis or breakdown of red blood cells) or the high level is related to the liver's inability to pick up the bilirubin (Gilbert's syndrome; (American Gastroenterological Association, 2002; Fiellin, Reid, & O'Connor, 2000; Friedman, 2015; Pratt & Kaplan, 2000). In the case of high direct levels of bilirubin, or conjugated bilirubin, there is a decrease in the removal of bile. Usually, this occurs in hepatobiliary diseases and certain genetic disorders (including Dubin–Johnson syndrome or Rotor's syndrome; American Gastroenterological Association, 2002; Fiellin, Reid, & O'Connor, 2000; Friedman, 2015; Pratt & Kaplan, 2000).

There are certain medications that can cause acute elevations in LFT readings. Some of those include nonsteroidal anti-inflammatory drugs (NSAIDS), acetaminophen, certain antibiotics, antiseizure medications, antituberculosis medications, antilipid agents (statins), sulfonylureas (glipizide), herbal medications (Chinese herbs and senna), and illicit drugs (including anabolic steroids, Ecstasy, and cocaine; American Gastroenterological Association, 2002; Fiellin, Reid, & O'Connor, 2000; Friedman, 2015; Pratt & Kaplan, 2000).

As mentioned, pregnancy can cause elevations of alkaline phosphatase and other liver enzymes. HELLP syndrome can occur in pregnancy; it stands for hemolysis, elevated liver enzymes, low platelets, and fatty liver of pregnancy. In cases of HELLP, liver failure is imminent and safe delivery of the baby is a priority to save the mother's life. Expert consultation is necessary, and the patient may need urgent transfer to a liver transplant center if her symptoms do not improve postpartum (Friedman, 2015).

Acute liver failure is rare, but can be a cause of abnormal LFT results. It is defined as LFT readings greater than 10 times the normal levels, hepatic encephalopathy (ranging from confusion and disorientation to coma), and a prolonged PT/INR level. If diagnosed, the patient with acute liver failure should be transferred immediately to a transplant center for urgent evaluation for a liver transplant (American Gastroenterological

Association, 2002; Fiellin, Reid, & O'Connor, 2000; Friedman, 2015; Pratt & Kaplan, 2000).

Other liver disease diagnoses that can cause elevations of LFT readings include autoimmune hepatitis (described in Chapter 19), viral hepatitis (described in Chapter 17), fatty liver disease (described in Chapter 18), hemochromatosis, Wilson's disease, and alpha-1 antitrypsin disease, which are described in more detail in Chapter 16. Other differential diagnoses to include are celiac disease, strenuous exercise, muscle disorders, and thyroid disorders (Friedman, 2015).

MANAGEMENT

If there is no evidence of liver failure or decompensation, the patient is asymptomatic, and there are no other laboratory abnormalities, repeat testing is recommended in 6 months. Any new medication that may have contributed to the abnormal testing should be stopped. Patients who are diabetic should try to optimize their treatment regimen to better control blood sugars. Patients should not drink alcohol and should make lifestyle modifications, including regular exercise and dietary changes to include more fruits and vegetables. If the repeat LFTs remain elevated after 6 months, patients should have an ultrasound and seek expert consultation (American Gastro-enterological Association, 2002; Fiellin, Reid, & O'Connor, 2000; Friedman, 2015; Pratt & Kaplan, 2000).

Expert consultation should be obtained for any patient with unexplained persistently abnormal LFT results and/or acute liver failure. Liver biopsy usually is required and should be performed by a highly trained expert (Friedman, 2015).

ICD-10 CODE

Abnormal results of liver function studies: R94.5
Abnormal findings on diagnostic imaging of liver and biliary tract: R93.2
Abnormal coagulation profile: R79.1

1. Abnormal LFT results are caused by disease, infection, drugs, or pregnancy.
2. An elevated INR is a red flag that an acute liver injury has occurred.
3. A thorough history is important to determine whether environmental factors or medications are to blame for LFT abnormalities.
4. Expert consultation should be obtained for any patient with unexplained persistent abnormal LFT results and/or acute liver failure.

REFERENCES

American Gastroenterological Association. (2002). American Gastroenterological Association medical position statement: Evaluation of liver chemistry tests. *Gastroenterology, 123,* 1364–1384.

Fiellin, D. A., Reid, M. C., & O'Connor, P. G. (2000). Outpatient management of patients with alcohol problems. *Annuals of Internal Medicine, 133,* 815–827.

Friedman, L. (2015). Approach to the patient with abnormal liver biochemical and function tests. Retrieved from www.uptodate.com/contents/approach-to-the-patient-with-abnormal-liver-biochemical-and-function-tests?source=search_result&search=Approach+to+the+patient+with+abnormal+liver&selectedTitle=1%7E150.

Pratt, D. S., & Kaplan, M. M. (2000). Evaluation of abnormal liver-enzyme results in asymptomatic patients. *New England Journal of Medicine, 342,* 1266–1271.

Sicklick, J. K., D'Angelica, M., & Fong, Y. (2012). The liver. In C. M. Townsend, R. D. Beauchamp, B. M. Evers, & K. L. Mattox (Eds.), *Sabiston textbook of surgery* (19th ed., pp. 1411–1475) Philadelphia, PA: Elsevier.

16

Causes of Liver Disease

This chapter focuses on the not-so-common causes of liver disease, including alpha-1 antitrypsin deficiency, Budd–Chiari syndrome (BCS), hemochromatosis, primary sclerosing cholangitis (PSC), primary biliary cirrhosis (PBC), polycystic liver disease, and Wilson's disease. Certain medications, such as isoniazid and methotrexate, have been known to cause hepatotoxicity. Infections can cause liver failure as well, including schistosomiasis, echinococcosis, syphilis, and brucellosis (Goldberg & Chopra, 2015). More common causes, including viral hepatitis, autoimmune hepatitis, and fatty liver disease (alcoholic and nonalcoholic), are discussed in future chapters.

At the end of this chapter, the reader will be able to:

1. Discuss the treatment for hemochromatosis
2. State the difference between primary sclerosing cholangitis and primary biliary cirrhosis
3. Name a classic diagnostic finding for Wilson's disease

CAUSES OF LIVER DISEASE

Genetic Disorders

Alpha-1 antitrypsin deficiency is a genetic abnormality that occurs in one in 2,000 individuals and indicates a problem with protein secretion. In most patients with this disorder, pulmonary disease is exhibited. There is no clinical presentation that is classic of alpha-1 antitrypsin deficiency. When patients present with liver issues, testing for this disorder is useful. Prognosis depends on the severity of disease in the liver or lungs. There is no definite medical treatment; however, liver transplant will cure the disease (Bacon, 2015).

Hereditary hemochromatosis (HH) is a genetic disorder from the mutation of the *HFE* (*human factors engineering*) protein, which causes increased iron absorption from the gut, creating an overload of iron in the pancreas, heart, and liver (Bacon, 2015).

Wilson's disease is a genetic autosomal recessive disorder seen in young patients, usually in adolescence. Approximately one in 30,000 individuals is affected. The disorder causes copper to accumulate in the liver, leading to hepatotoxicity. Other areas affected include the eyes, joints, red blood cells, and kidneys (Bacon, 2015). In 5% of patients with Wilson's disease, acute liver failure occurs (Schilsky, 2014).

Polycystic liver disease is also an inherited condition that may or may not be seen with polycystic kidney disease. Diagnosis is made by imaging studies when 20 or more cysts in the liver are identified. Women are more likely to have the disease, and age of onset of symptoms is usually in the 30s or 40s. It causes progressive enlargement of the liver, and patients can have severe hepatomegaly that is incapacitating (Khan, Dennison, & Garcea, 2016).

Vascular Disorders

Vascular disorders of the liver include congenital vascular malformations, portal vein thrombosis, sinusoidal obstruction syndrome, and BCS (DeLeve, Valla, & Garcia-Tsao, 2009). The

American Association for the Study of Liver Disease (AASLD) has provided guidelines for managing these vascular disorders. This chapter focuses on BCS. It is a disorder in which the blood flow out of the liver is obstructed, usually by thrombosis of one or all of the hepatic veins or the inferior vena cava (DeLeve et al., 2009; Torres & Paredes, 2015). It can be secondary, meaning it is caused by compression from tumor (benign or malignant), or primary, in which it is caused by phlebitis or thrombosis. Factors that contribute to the development of BCS are those that cause a hypercoagulable state, such as clotting factor deficiencies (possibly from an inherited disorder), malignancy, recent pregnancy, or oral contraceptive use (DeLeve et al., 2009).

Biliary Diseases

Primary sclerosing cholangitis (PSC) is a chronic biliary disorder that affects the bile ducts, causing inflammation, fibrosis, and, eventually, biliary strictures. It is more common in men, with onset at 40 years of age (Eaton, Talwalkar, & LaRusso, 2015). Imaging studies, specifically endoscopic retrograde cholangiopancreatography (ERCP), show bile duct changes of strictures and dilatations. The most common laboratory abnormality is an elevation of alkaline phosphatase. There is a strong association with PSC and inflammatory bowel disease (IBD), typically ulcerative colitis. These patients also have a higher risk of developing cholangiocarcinoma (Chapman et al., 2010). When biliary strictures occur, complications can result, including cholangitis and sepsis. When these issues become recurrent, liver transplantation may be indicated.

PBC is an autoimmune disorder that affects the bile ducts. Women are more affected than men, with onset in the 40s to 50s (Eaton et al., 2015). A serologic marker that is highly suggestive of PBC is antimitochondrial antibody (AMA). It is a chronic disorder, taking sometimes decades for complications to develop. Diagnosis is determined by elevation of alkaline phosphatase levels, manifestation of AMA, and destruction of bile ducts seen on liver biopsy. Approximately a third of patients with PBC have a higher tendency toward osteoporosis (Lindor et al., 2009).

ASSESSMENT FINDINGS

Alpha-1 antitrypsin deficiency with liver involvement may not show symptoms until chronic liver disease is present. If lung involvement is present, emphysema is noted; and this is worsened by smoking (Bacon, 2015).

Hemochromatosis can cause symptoms, including grayish or bronzed skin, enlarged liver (hepatomegaly), possible cirrhosis, tenderness and/or swelling of the second and third metacarpophalangeal joints, and weakness and fatigue. Most patients are asymptomatic and diagnosis is made after routine testing shows abnormal iron studies (Bacon, 2015).

Wilson's disease can cause several physical findings, including tremor, Kayser–Fleischer rings (classic ophthalmologic finding), hemolytic anemia, and arthropathy (Bacon, 2015).

Polycystic liver disease can cause severe hepatomegaly, abdominal distension, loss of appetite, malnutrition, and can have a huge impact on quality of life. Liver cysts can develop complications, including infection and hemorrhage, or can push on other abdominal structures such as the portal vein, inferior vena cava, or biliary system (Khan et al., 2016).

BCS should be considered in patients with abdominal pain, hepatomegaly, ascites, or with known risk factors of thrombosis (use of hormones, history of malignancy, recent pregnancy, etc.; DeLeve et al., 2009).

Patients with PBC may be asymptomatic or may have symptoms that include pruritus, fatigue, and sicca syndrome. Jaundice may be present, but is usually a late finding of disease (Lindor et al., 2009). Patients with PSC may develop biliary strictures, and this may be complicated by cholangitis and sepsis. Close monitoring for fever, chills, and other signs of sepsis is important.

PERTINENT LABORATORY FINDINGS

Routine laboratory testing, including complete blood count, complete metabolic panel, liver profile, and coagulation studies, is performed in patients with suspected liver disease.

Patients with hemochromatosis will have elevated iron studies. Iron studies tested are serum iron, total iron-binding capacity (TIBC) or transferrin, and serum ferritin. If the results of the iron studies are abnormal, genetic testing should be performed. Liver biopsy can be performed to determine the degree of liver damage from the iron overload (Bacon, 2015).

The screening test for Wilson's disease is determination of a ceruloplasmin level. If this level is abnormal, a 24-hour copper urine level should be obtained (Bacon, 2015).

There is no screening test for polycystic liver disease. Abnormal laboratory testing may include an increased tumor marker (CA 19-9), gamma-glutamyltransferase, and alkaline phosphate (Khan et al., 2016).

A hematologist consultation is recommended for the patient with BCS to evaluate for clotting disorders. Usually the patient with BCS has one or more inherited clotting disorder that has predisposed the blood clots to form. Ultrasonography is performed to evaluate the hepatic vasculature for thrombosis or blood-flow issues (DeLeve et al., 2009). The gold standard for evaluating the hepatic veins is hepatic venography (Torres & Paredes, 2015).

There can be some laboratory abnormalities in patients with PSC and PBC. These include mild alkaline phosphatase, alanine aminotransferase (ALT), and aspartate aminotransferase (AST). With PBC, there is some association with the severity of bile duct issues and elevation of alkaline phosphatase levels. There may also be an elevation of cholesterol levels (Lindor et al., 2009).

MANAGEMENT

Treatment for the patient with hemochromatosis includes phlebotomy weekly or twice a week, removing one unit of whole blood. Most of the time, liver enzyme abnormalities resolve with treatment and patients do not have complications. If cirrhosis has developed, however, phlebotomy will not improve symptoms (Bacon, 2015). Vitamin C should be avoided because of the potential to cause increased free radical activity in patients with high iron levels (Bacon, Adams, Kowdley, Powell, & Tavill, 2011).

Wilson's disease management includes D-penicillamine and trientine, which are copper-chelating drugs. Zinc supplementation is also used in treatment for prevention of reaccumulation of copper. Liver transplantation will cure disease (Bacon, 2015; Roberts & Schilsky, 2008; Schilsky, 2014).

There are some medications that can help reduce the size of the cysts in polycystic liver disease. Some options are somatostatin classes, including lanreotide and octreotide, or immunosuppressive agents, including everolimus and sirolimus. Surgical options are available for patients with debilitating effects, such as liver resection, removal of cysts, and liver transplantation (Khan et al., 2016).

For patients with BCS, anticoagulation therapy is recommended and will likely be needed indefinitely unless contraindicated. If there are other causes of liver disease, these must be managed as well. Patients may meet criteria for liver transplantation if complications of liver failure arise. Patients should be referred to a transplant center for evaluation and close monitoring (DeLeve et al., 2009).

Management for patients with PBC includes ursodeoxycholic acid (UDCA) in a dose of 13 to 15 mg/kg/day by mouth. Pruritus is common in patients with PBC and is often difficult to manage. Options include bile acid sequestrants, opiate antagonists, and sertraline. It is important to check for osteoporosis and ensure vitamin deficiencies are corrected. If complications of liver disease arise, then liver transplantation remains an option (Lindor et al., 2009).

There is no approved medication for management of PSC, although use of UDCA has been studied.

ICD-10 CODE

Alpha-1 antitrypsin deficiency: E88.01
Budd–Chiari syndrome: I82.0
Hemochromatosis, other: E83.118
Hemochromatosis, unspecified: E83.119
Hereditary hemochromatosis: E83.110
Primary sclerosing cholangitis: K83.0

Primary biliary cirrhosis: K74.3
Polycystic liver disease (cystic disease of the liver): Q44.6
Wilson's disease: E83.01

======= *FAST FACTS in a NUTSHELL*

1. Phlebotomy is recommended for patients with hemo-chromatosis to control iron levels.
2. PSC and PBC are both chronic biliary disorders.
3. There is an association between PSC and IBD.
4. Classic physical examination findings of Wilson's disease include Kayser–Fleischer rings.
5. Lifelong anticoagulation is usually needed for patients with BCS.
6. Any cause of liver disease can result in liver failure or cirrhosis. Referral to a specialist at a transplant center is recommended to appropriately manage these disorders.

REFERENCES

Bacon, B. R. (2015). Inheritable forms of liver disease. In P. R. McNally (Ed.), *GI/liver secrets plus* (5th ed., pp. 243–249). Philadelphia, PA: Elsevier Saunders.

Bacon, B. R., Adams, P. C., Kowdley, K. V., Powell, L. W., & Tavill, A. S. (2011). Diagnosis and management of hemochromatosis: 2011 Practice guideline by the American Association for the Study of Liver Diseases. *Hepatology, 54*(1), 328–343.

Chapman, R., Fevery, J., Kalloo, A., Nagorney, D. M., Boberg, K. M., Shneider, B., & Gores, G. J. (2010). Diagnosis and management of primary sclerosing cholangitis. *Hepatology, 51*(2), 660–678.

DeLeve, L. D., Valla, D., & Garcia-Tsao, G. (2009). Vascular disorders of the liver. *Hepatology, 49,* 1729–1764.

Eaton, J. E., Talwalkar, J. A., & LaRusso, N. F. (2015). Primary biliary cirrhosis and primary sclerosing cholangitis. In P. R. McNally (Ed.), *GI/liver secrets plus* (5th ed., pp. 146–154). Philadelphia, PA: Elsevier Saunders.

Goldberg, E., & Chopra, S. (2015). Cirrhosis in adults: Etiologies, clinical manifestations, and diagnosis. Retrieved from www .uptodate.com/contents/cirrhosis-in-adults-etiologies-clinical-manifestations-and-diagnosis?source=search_result&search=Cirrh osis+in+adults%3A+Etiologies%2C&selectedTitle=1%7E150.html

Khan, S., Dennison, A., & Garcea, G. (2016). Medical therapy for polycystic liver disease. *Annals of the Royal College of Surgeons of England, 98,* 18–23.

Lindor, K. D., Gershwin, E., Poupon, R., Kaplan, M., Bergasa, N. V., & Heathcote, E. J. (2009). Primary biliary cirrhosis. *Hepatology, 50*(1), 291–308.

Roberts, E. A., & Schilsky, M. L. (2008). Diagnosis and treatment of Wilson disease: An update. *Hepatology, 47*(6), 2089–2111.

Schilsky, M. L. (2014). Wilson disease: Clinical manifestations, diagnosis, and treatment. *Clinical Liver Disease, 3*(5), 104–107.

Torres, D. M., & Paredes, A. H. (2015). Vascular liver disease. In P. R. McNally (Ed.), *GI/liver secrets plus* (5th ed., pp. 202–209). Philadelphia, PA: Elsevier Saunders.

17

Viral Hepatitis

Viral hepatitis *is defined as an inflammatory response to a virus that has infected hepatocytes, or liver cells. Viral hepatitis includes hepatitis A, B, C, D, and E; these viruses reproduce in the hepatocytes. If the immune system is strong enough to attack the infection aggressively, severe liver injury can occur causing acute liver failure. More common, especially with hepatitis B and C, gradual injury occurs, causing chronic liver disease, sometimes progressing to cirrhosis or hepatocellular carcinoma.*

At the end of this chapter, the reader will be able to:

1. Name which types of hepatitis are transmitted via fecal–oral route and which are transmitted via blood or body fluid routes
2. State three signs and symptoms associated with an acute viral hepatitis infection
3. Name two new medications available to treat hepatitis C

TYPES OF VIRAL HEPATITIS

Hepatitis A is a viral infection transmitted via the fecal–oral route. Risk factors for infection include exposure to poor sanitary conditions, travel to endemic areas, ingestion of contaminated food or water, low socioeconomic status, and crowded living conditions. Half of Americans have antibodies by age 50. Once exposed, patients will have lifelong immunity, exhibited by the antibody in the bloodstream (antibodies to hepatitis A virus [anti-HAV]) and diagnosis is made by positive anti-HAV immunoglobulin M (IgM) testing. There is an incubation period of 2 to 6 weeks (Kumar, Abbas, & Aster, 2014).

The hepatitis B virus (HBV) affects more than 2 billion people in the world, with over 1 million Americans having chronic hepatitis B. Areas endemic with this virus are Asia, Africa, the Western Pacific, the Middle East, the Arctic, some areas of South America, and Eastern Europe (Kumar et al., 2014). This is the most common viral hepatitis to cause an acute response in patients. It is transmitted by exposure to contaminated blood and body fluids, most often through injection drug use. Other modes of transmission include perinatal and sexual transmission, as well as exposure from hemodialysis. Risk factors include men who have sex with men, health care workers, body piercing or tattoo recipients, travel to endemic areas, having received a blood transfusion prior to 1992, immunosuppressed patients, and living with a person with HBV. Patients can be coinfected with hepatitis D virus or HIV (Teo & Lok, 2014). One to 2% of patients progress to chronic infection (Lok & McMahon, 2009).

The hepatitis C virus (HCV) affects more than 3.6 million Americans, and over 170 million people worldwide (Kumar et al., 2014). Patients at particularly high risk for HCV infection include individuals who use or have used intravenous drugs, intranasal drugs, who have hemodialysis, who have been incarcerated, who are health care workers, children born to HCV-positive mothers, and individuals who received a blood transfusion or organ/tissue transplant before 1992. In the United States, injection-drug use is blamed for approximately 60% of acute infections of HCV. The U.S. Preventive Services Task Force (USPSTF) and the Centers for Disease Control (CDC) recommend a one-time HCV test or screening for patients who were born between 1945 and 1965. It is also recommended that individuals who meet one or more of the high-risk criteria undergo screening as well (American Association for the Study of Liver Disease [AASLD] & Infectious Diseases Society of America [ISDA], 2016).

The hepatitis D virus (HDV) is called a satellite virus; it must have HBV in the system to survive. There are two forms of this infection. One is coinfection, in which there is HBV and HDV infection simultaneously. The second is called *superinfection,* in which HDV is superimposed on chronic HBV infection, causing an acute flare of hepatitis. The mode of transmission for HDV infection is the same as HBV infection (Hanson, Pearson, & Kugelmas, 2015). It is seen mostly in the Mediterranean countries, and rarely in the United States (Lok & McMahon, 2009).

The hepatitis E virus (HEV) is similar to HAV in its transmission modes and in that infection is usually acute. It is prevalent in India, Asia, Central America, and developing countries. Infection with HEV can be fatal for pregnant women (Hanson et al., 2015).

PERTINENT LABORATORY FINDINGS

Abnormal laboratory findings for the patient with acute hepatitis include acute elevation of alanine transaminase/aspartate aminotransferase (ALT/AST), hypoglycemia, coagulopathy (elevated international normalized ratio [INR]), hypoalbuminemia, hyponatremia, pancytopenia (anemia, leukopenia, and thrombocytopenia), as well as acute kidney injury (Hanson et al., 2015). For tests for acute hepatitis infection, see Table 17.1.

As mentioned, the HCV screening test is recommended for certain individuals. If the screening test is positive, HCV

TABLE 17.1 Viral Hepatitis Testing

Hepatitis Type	Testing for Acute Disease	Testing for Chronic Disease
A	IgM anti-HAV (antibody to HAV)	None
B	IgM anti-HBc (core antibody), initially and then replaced by IgG anti-HBc	HBsAg (first marker to appear)
	May have elevated aminotransferase levels	HBeAg and HBV DNA (can show active replication)
	HBV DNA (can show acute infection)	HBeAg with HBV DNA will determine whether chronic hepatitis B is present and guide treatment
	HBsAg (can also indicate chronic infection)	
C	HCV RNA (sensitive within 10 days of exposure)	Anti-HCV
	Anti-HCV (may be negative early)	
D	IgG and IgM anti-HDV, HDV RNA	Total anti-HDV
E	IgG and IgM anti-HEV, HEV RNA	None

Anti-HAV, hepatitis A antibody; anti-HBc, hepatitis B core antigen; anti-HCV, hepatitis C antibody; anti-HDV, hepatitis D antibody; anti-HEV, hepatitis E antibody; HBeAg, hepatitis B envelope antigen; HBsAg, hepatitis B surface antigen; HBV DNA, hepatitis B viral load; HCV RNA, hepatitis C viral load; IgG, immunoglobulin G; IgM, immunoglobulin M.
Source: Cutler (2013)

ribonucleic acid (RNA) measurement should be obtained to confirm and assess viral load.

ASSESSMENT

In patients with viral hepatitis, signs and symptoms can vary greatly, ranging from asymptomatic to acute liver failure. Patients may complain of nausea, vomiting, decreased appetite, generalized malaise, fever, jaundice, dark or tea-colored urine, abdominal pain to the right upper quadrant, or clay-colored or light stools. On examination, providers may note hepatomegaly (Hanson et al., 2015).

The best initial imaging study used to visualize the liver is ultrasound. Other possible testing may include a liver biopsy to evaluate the extent of liver damage (Hanson et al., 2015).

DIFFERENTIAL DIAGNOSIS

The differential diagnosis when considering viral hepatitis may include the following:

- Acute infections such as Epstein–Barr virus or cytomegalovirus (CMV), yellow fever, toxoplasmosis, malaria, Q fever, syphilis, adenovirus
- Drug toxicity and/or poisoning
- Hemolytic diseases
- Hepatocellular carcinoma
- Acute cholangitis
- Sepsis
- Autoimmune hepatitis
- Ischemic liver injury
- Alcoholic hepatitis

MANAGEMENT

Supportive therapy is recommended for the management of acute viral hepatitis. To prevent further liver damage, patients should be instructed to avoid alcohol consumption as well as acetaminophen. In certain cases of acute HCV infection, patients may clear virus independent of antiviral therapy. To avoid transmission of HAV and HEV, food-safety techniques and proper sanitation/hygiene measures are important. Individuals should not eat or drink tap water when traveling to areas endemic with these types of infections. Vaccinations for hepatitis A and B are available and are recommended for patients who meet high-risk criteria. Patients with viral hepatitis should be educated on modes of transmission, possible treatment options, and cost of antiviral medications (if indicated). It is recommended that family members be vaccinated. In cases of hepatitis B, C, or D, referral to a specialist is warranted. Rarely does acute liver failure occur, and urgent evaluation at a transplant center is recommended.

Chronic viral hepatitis usually develops in patients with hepatitis B and/or C infection. The goals of treatment for patients with hepatitis B are to stop viral replication, attain normal liver function, and prevent progression to cirrhosis or hepatocellular carcinoma. The goal for hepatitis C treatment is to cure the disease, which is also known as a *sustained viral response* or SVR (undetectable HCV level for at least 12 weeks; Hanson et al., 2015). There are many new hepatitis C medications available, with an over 90% cure rate. These medications are costly; however, the pharmaceutical and insurance companies are making attempts to make them affordable so patients can be treated. The treatment of hepatitis C is mainly by oral medications only (no more need for interferon, which had many adverse, undesired effects for patients). See Table 17.2 for hepatitis C management options. New medications are coming on to the market that are universal in treating all genotypes.

TABLE 17.2 Updated Hepatitis C Treatment Strategies for Treatment of Naive Patients*

	Treatment Options		
Genotype (Type of Virus)	Without Cirrhosis	With Compensated Cirrhosis	With Decompensated Cirrhosis*
1a and 1b	Treatment naive: • Elbasvir 50 mg/ grazoprevir 100 mg (Zepratier) daily for 12 weeks • Ledipasvir 90 mg/ sofosbuvir 400 mg (Harvoni) daily for 12 weeks	Treatment naive (1a): • Elbasvir 50 mg/ grazoprevir 100 mg (Zepratier) daily for 12 weeks • Ledipasvir 90 mg/ sofosbuvir 400 mg (Harvoni) daily for 12 weeks	• Ledipasvir 90 mg/ sofosbuvir 400 mg (Harvoni) daily + low-dose RBV (600 mg) for 12 weeks OR

(continued)

	Treatment Options		
Genotype (Type of Virus)	**Without Cirrhosis**	**With Compensated Cirrhosis**	**With Decompensated Cirrhosis****
1a and 1b	• Paritaprevir 150 mg/ritonavir 100 mg/ombitasvir 25 mg daily + dasabuvir 250 mg (Viekira Pak ®) twice a day with weight based ribavirin (RBV) for 12 weeks (type 1b – same treatment as above, but without RBV) • Simeprevir 150 mg (Olysio) daily + sofosbuvir (Sovaldi) 400 mg daily for 12 weeks • Daclatasvir 60 mg (Daklinza) daily + sofosbuvir 400 mg (Sovaldi) daily for 12 weeks	Treatment naive (1b): • Elbasvir 50 mg/ grazoprevir 100 mg (Zepratier) daily for 12 weeks • Ledipasvir 90 mg/ sofosbuvir 400 mg (Harvoni) daily for 12 weeks • Paritaprevir 150 mg/ ritonavir 100 mg/ ombitasvir 25 mg daily + dasabuvir 250 mg (Viekira Pak) twice a day for 12 weeks	• Daclatasvir 60 mg (Daklinza) daily + sofosbuvir 400 mg (Sovaldi) daily + low dose RBV (600 mg) for 12 weeks If unable to tolerate RBV: • Ledipasvir 90 mg/ sofosbuvir 400 mg (Harvoni) daily + low-dose RBV (600 mg) for 24 weeks • Daclatasvir 60 mg (Daklinza) daily + sofosbuvir 400 mg (Sovaldi) daily for 24 weeks
2	• Sofosbuvir (Sovaldi) 400 mg daily + weight-based RBV for 12 weeks • Daclatasvir 60 mg (Daklinza) daily + sofosbuvir 400 mg (Sovaldi) daily for 12 weeks (for those who cannot take RBV)	• Sofosbuvir (Sovaldi) 400 mg daily + weight-based RBV for 16–24 weeks • Daclatasvir 60 mg (Daklinza) daily + sofosbuvir 400 mg (Sovaldi) daily for 16–24 weeks (for those who cannot take RBV)	• Daclatasvir 60 mg (Daklinza) daily + sofosbuvir 400 mg (Sovaldi) daily + low-dose RBV (600 mg) for 12 weeks

(*continued*)

TABLE 17.2 Updated Hepatitis C Treatment Strategies for Treatment of Naive Patients (Continued)

	Treatment Options		
Genotype (Type of Virus)	Without Cirrhosis	With Compensated Cirrhosis	With Decompensated Cirrhosis*
3	• Daclatasvir 60 mg (Daklinza) daily + sofosbuvir 400 mg (Sovaldi) daily for 12 weeks • Sofosbuvir (Sovaldi) 400 mg daily + weight-based RBV + weekly PEG-IFN for 12 weeks	• Daclatasvir 60 mg (Daklinza) daily + sofosbuvir 400 mg (Sovaldi) daily for 24 weeks with or without weight-based RBV • Sofosbuvir (Sovaldi) 400 mg daily + weight-based RBV + weekly PEG-IFN for 12 weeks (suitable to take interferon)	• Same as genotype 2
4	Paritaprevir 150 mg/ritonavir 100 mg/ ombitasvir 25 mg daily (Technivie) + weight-based RBV for 12 weeks Elbasvir 50 mg/grazoprevir 100 mg (Zepratier) daily for 12 weeks Ledipasvir 90 mg/sofosbuvir 400 mg (Harvoni) daily for 12 weeks		• Same as genotype 1
5 6	Ledipasvir 90 mg/sofosbuvir 400 mg (Harvoni) daily for 12 weeks		

*Should be referred to a specialist, ideally a liver transplant center.
RBV, ribavirin; PEG-IFN, pegylated interferon.
**As of July 2016. For latest treatment recommendation please go to www .hcvguidelines.org
Source: AASLD and IDSA (2016).

ICD-10 CODE

Hepatitis A without hepatic coma: B15.9
Acute hepatitis B without delta-agent and without hepatic coma: B16.9
Other specified acute viral hepatitis: B17.8
Acute viral hepatitis, unspecified: B17.9

Chronic viral hepatitis B with delta agent: B18.0
Chronic viral hepatitis B without delta agent: B18.1
Chronic viral hepatitis C: B18.2
Chronic viral hepatitis, unspecified: B18.9
Carrier of viral hepatitis B: Z22.51
Carrier of viral hepatitis C: Z22.52

―――――――――――*FAST FACTS in a NUTSHELL*

1. It is not recommended that antivirals be used to treat acute viral hepatitis.
2. The USPSTF and CDC recommend a one-time screening test for HCV (antibody HCV) for all patients who were born between 1945 and 1965 and for individuals who meet high-risk criteria.
3. A *sustained virologic response,* or *virologic cure,* is defined as an undetectable HCV RNA level for at least 12 weeks.
4. Acute hepatitis infection can progress to chronic hepatitis.
5. All patients with viral hepatitis should be instructed to abstain from alcohol and acetaminophen use.
6. In cases of hepatitis B, C, or D, referral to a specialist is warranted. Urgent evaluation at a transplant center is recommended for patients with acute liver failure.

REFERENCES

American Association for the Study of Liver Disease (AASLD) & Infectious Diseases Society of America (IDSA). (2016). Recommendations for testing, managing, and treating hepatitis C. Retrieved from www.hcvguidelines.org/

Cutler, N. (2013). Understanding hepatitis B serology. Retrieved from www.hepatitiscentral.com/news/understanding-hepatitis-b-serology/

Hanson, C., Pearson, G., & Kugelmas, M. (2015). General concepts on viral hepatitis. In P. R. McNally (Ed.), *GI/liver secrets plus* (5th ed., pp. 101–105). Philadelphia, PA: Elsevier Saunders.

Kumar, V., Abbas, A., & Aster, J. C. (2014). *Robbins & Cotran: Pathologic basis of disease* (9th ed.). St. Louis, MO: Elsevier.

Lok, A.S. & McMahon, B.J. (2009). Chronic hepatitis B: Update 2009. Hepatology, 50(3), 661-662

Teo, E., & Lok, A. (2014). Epidemiology, transmission, and prevention of hepatitis B virus infection. Retrieved from www.uptodate.com/contents/epidemiology-transmission-and-prevention-of-hepatitis-b-virus-infection?source=search_result&search=Epidemiology%2C+transmission%2C+and+prevention&selectedTitle=1%7E150.html

18

Fatty Liver Disease

Fatty liver disease is a broad term used to describe both alcoholic liver disease (ALD) and nonalcoholic fatty liver disease (NAFLD). Both types of fatty liver disease are becoming increasingly common, especially NAFLD. This chapter briefly discusses both types.

At the end of this chapter, the reader will be able to:

1. Distinguish between ALD and NAFLD
2. Define four risk factors for developing nonalcoholic steatohepatitis (NASH)
3. Name four nonpharmacologic treatments for managing NASH

ALCOHOLIC VERSUS NONALCOHOLIC FATTY LIVER DISEASE

ALD includes a wide range of liver injury from simple fatty infiltration into liver cells, to alcoholic hepatitis, fibrosis and cirrhosis. There are some possible risk factors that may increase the risk of liver injury when consuming alcohol. They include the type, amount, and duration of alcohol consumption, being female, African American or Hispanic ancestry, history of binge drinking, and other comorbid conditions, including viral hepatitis, obesity, and hemochromatosis. There is a high mortality rate, with over 40% of deaths from liver disease linked to alcohol consumption. Mortality is increased if malnutrition exists as well. Diagnosis is made by history of significant alcohol intake, associated laboratory data, and indications of liver disease on physical examination and imaging studies (O'Shea et al., 2010).

The American Association for the Study of Liver Disease (AASLD) Practice Guideline defines *NAFLD* as hepatic steatosis (seen on imaging or on liver biopsy), and exclusion of all other possible reasons for hepatic steatosis (e.g., alcohol, genetic, and medication causes) Chalasani et al., 2012. Like ALD, NAFLD encompasses a large spectrum of disease progression, from simple fatty infiltration of the liver cells to NASH, hepatocellular carcinoma (HCC), and/or cirrhosis. Risk factors associated with the development of NAFLD include metabolic syndrome, type 2 diabetes mellitus, hypertension, coronary artery disease, hypertriglyceridemia, and obesity. Hispanic individuals, those older than 45, and people with a significant family history of fatty liver disease, metabolic syndrome, or cardiovascular disease are at higher risk. NAFLD has become one of the most common causes of liver disease, with a worldwide prevalence of 20% (Chaney, 2015).

ASSESSMENT FINDINGS

It is important to thoroughly review the patient's alcohol consumption history. ALD is associated with consumption of more than 35 units of alcohol per week (1 unit=10 to 12 g; Drinane & Shah, 2013). The CAGE questionnaire is a useful tool used to further investigate whether alcoholism is an issue. Other associated comorbidities or risk factors are noted in the patient's history. Patients may complain of yellowing of skin or eyes, itching, or right upper quadrant abdominal pain. Dietary history and lifestyle choices should be reviewed. Social history is obtained and includes use of illicit drugs or intravenous drug use, prior history of blood transfusions (particularly if prior to 1992), and sexual activity (Chaney, 2015).

On physical examination, patients with fatty liver disease may be asymptomatic. Some physical signs that may be present for ALD include gynecomastia, Dupuytren's contracture, and parotid enlargement. Signs of progression to cirrhosis include ascites, veins that are seen on the abdomen, hepatic encephalopathy, and edema (O'Shea et al., 2010). The patient with NASH may have dorsocervicallipohypertrophy. There may be liver or spleen enlargement if chronic liver disease is present (Chaney, 2015).

PERTINENT LABORATORY FINDINGS

A classic laboratory finding for the patient with ALD is aspartate aminotransferase (AST) levels two times greater than alanine transaminase (ALT) levels, usually a 2:1 ratio. Other laboratory findings include hypoalbuminemia, elevated ferritin levels, elevated triglycerides, and thrombocytopenia. Alcoholic hepatitis is associated with elevations of alkaline phosphatase, gamma-glutamyltranspeptidase, and hyperbilirubinemia. Poor nutrition is associated with elevation of mean corpuscular volume seen on complete blood count (Kulig, 2015). Other testing includes hemoglobin (Hgb) A1C, lipid panel, and viral hepatitis serologies.

The NAFLD fibrosis score is a useful tool used to predict fibrosis by means of age, platelet count, certain laboratory values, body mass index (BMI), and presence of diabetes or glucose intolerance (Chaney, 2015).

IMAGING STUDIES

Several imaging studies useful to assess for fatty liver include ultrasound, CT scan, or MRI. Liver biopsy may be needed to determine the degree of liver injury. Pathology reports commonly note Mallory hyaline on liver biopsy with fatty liver disease (Kulig, 2015).

There is no screening test available for NAFLD, and routine screening is not recommended (Chalasani et al., 2012).

MANAGEMENT

All patients with fatty liver disease should abstain from alcohol. For patients with alcoholism, a formal support system such as Alcoholics Anonymous is important. Commonly, nutrition deficits, including malnutrition and vitamin deficiencies, coexist with fatty liver disease. Patients may need aggressive nutritional support to improve the condition. In cases of severe alcoholic hepatitis, prednisolone 40 mg daily for 28 days, followed by a tapering dose can be prescribed. If liver disease has progressed to cirrhosis, liver transplantation may be needed if the patient is a candidate (O'Shea et al., 2010).

Lifestyle modifications are the mainstay of treatment for patients with NAFLD. A 3% to 5% weight loss can improve liver disease (Chalasani et al., 2012). Recommendations include increasing exercise and dietary changes such as a low-fat, low-cholesterol diet, weight loss, and eliminating trans fats and high-fructose corn syrup. A support system is crucial for patients to be successful. Omega-3 fatty acids can be useful if patients have hypertriglyceridemia. Fat-soluble vitamin deficiencies are common in patients with liver disease and should be corrected by supplementations (Chaney, 2015).

ICD-10 CODE

Alcoholic liver disease, unspecified: K70.9
Alcoholic fatty liver: K70.0
Alcoholic cirrhosis of liver without ascites: K70.30
Alcoholic hepatic failure with coma: K70.41
Alcoholic hepatic failure without coma: K70.40
Alcoholic hepatitis with ascites: K70.11
Alcoholic hepatitis without ascites: K 70.10
Fatty (change of) liver, not elsewhere classified: K76.0
Nonalcoholic steatohepatitis (NASH): K75.81

1. A 2:1 ratio of AST to ALT is a common laboratory finding in patients with alcoholic liver disease.
2. Fatty liver disease and malnutrition commonly coexist.
3. Lifestyle modifications are the mainstay of treatment for patients with NAFLD.
4. Optimizing the patient's nutritional status is important for the patient with fatty liver disease.

REFERENCES

Chalasani, N., Younossi, Z., Lavine, J. E., Diehl, A. M., Brunt, E. M., Cusi, K., . . . Sanyal, A. J. (2012). The diagnosis and management of non-alcoholic fatty liver disease: Practice guideline by the American Association for the Study of Liver Diseases, and the American Gastroenterological Association. *Hepatology, 55*(6), 2005–2023.

Chaney, A. (2015). Treating the patient with non-alcoholic fatty liver disease. *Nurse Practitioner, 40*(11), 36–42.

Drinane, M. C., & Shah, V. H. (2013). Alcoholic hepatitis: Diagnosis and prognosis. *Clinical Liver Disease, 2*(2), 80–83.

Kulig, C. (2015). Alcoholic liver disease, alcoholism, and alcohol withdrawal syndrome. In P. R. McNally (Ed.), *GI/liver secrets plus* (5th ed., pp. 101–105). Philadelphia, PA: Elsevier Saunders.

O'Shea, R. S., Dasarathy, S., McCullough, A. J., & the Practice Guideline Committee of the American Association for the Study of Liver Diseases and the Practice Parameters Committee of the American College of Gastroenterology. (2010). Alcoholic liver disease. *Hepatology, 51*(1), 307–328.

19

Autoimmune Liver Disease

The American Association for the Study of Liver Disease (AASLD) defines autoimmune hepatitis (AIH) as an "unresolving inflammation of the liver of unknown cause" (Manns et al., 2010, p. 1). Diagnosis is made by documenting the presence of autoantibodies, abnormal histology and globulin levels, and certain abnormal laboratory data (Manns et al., 2010). There are two types of AIH. Type 1 is more common and is associated with the presence in the bloodstream of antinuclear antibodies (ANA), smooth muscle antibodies (SMA), or both. Testing for antibodies of liver/kidney microsome type 1 (LKM-1) is performed; this is associated with type 2 AIH and is more common in children (Manns et al., 2010). Women are more often diagnosed than men, usually prior to age 40. In one third of patients, other autoimmune diseases coexist, including Grave's disease, rheumatoid arthritis, synovitis, and ulcerative colitis (Czaja, 2015). As with other causes of liver disease, AIH can progress to cirrhosis and/or hepatocellular carcinoma.

At the end of this chapter, the reader will be able to:

1. Define autoimmune hepatitis
2. State two classic laboratory markers associated with a diagnosis of autoimmune hepatitis
3. Name two treatment options for treating autoimmune hepatitis

ASSESSMENT FINDINGS

A thorough history and physical examination should be performed. Other etiologies of liver disease should be investigated and excluded. Patients with autoimmune hepatitis may be asymptomatic, or complain of fatigue, generalized weakness, joint pains, nausea, jaundice, or abdominal pain (Czaja, 2015; Manns et al., 2010). Patients may also develop symptoms acutely, causing severe liver dysfunction.

PERTINENT LABORATORY FINDINGS

ANA and/or SMA are associated with autoimmune hepatitis; titer levels sometimes reach more than 1:80. Antimitochondrial antibody (AMA) testing is negative. Another classic finding is an elevated immunoglobulin G (IgG) level and hypergammaglobulinemia, more than 1.5 times the upper normal limit (Czaja, 2015; Manns et al., 2010). ALT and AST levels may be elevated. Viral hepatitis serologies usually are performed and are negative.

IMAGING STUDIES

Liver biopsy may be needed to evaluate the extent of liver injury and to evaluate for cirrhosis.

DIFFERENTIAL DIAGNOSIS

Differential diagnosis when considering the diagnosis of autoimmune hepatitis includes the following:

- Alcoholic liver disease
- Alpha-1 antitrypsin deficiency
- Celiac disease
- Chronic viral hepatitis

- Medication-related hepatitis (particularly nitrofurantoin and minocycline)
- Hemochromatosis
- Nonalcoholic steatohepatitis
- Primary biliary cirrhosis
- Primary sclerosing cholangitis
- Wilson's disease (Czaja, 2015; Lucey & Vierling, 2014).

MANAGEMENT

The AASLD recommends starting treatment for AIH with immunosuppression for those with liver injury. Consultation with an expert is required for further management. Patients are usually started on prednisone 30 mg daily and then tapered to 10 mg daily within 4 weeks, plus 50 mg daily of azathioprine (Manns et al., 2010). Patients may need stronger immunosuppression if first-line therapies fail. Other options include tacrolimus, mycophenolatemofetil, cyclosporine, sirolimus, antitumor necrosis factor (infliximab), and rituximab (Manns & Taubert, 2014). Because of the need for long-term immunosuppression, the patient with AIH needs to be monitored closely for bone disease (osteoporosis), as well as for signs of infection. Vaccination against hepatitis A and B, if not done already, is performed to prevent further liver injury. Lifestyle modifications to minimize risk of bone loss are recommended, such as weight-bearing exercises and consuming adequate calcium and vitamin D. Treatment with bisphosphates may be needed if osteoporosis is already present. Azathioprine has a pregnancy category D; and if pregnancy is considered or occurs, it should be stopped immediately (Manns et al., 2010). Patients should be followed up closely by a specialist (hepatologist). If acute deterioration of liver disease is noted, urgent liver transplant evaluation is warranted.

ICD-10 CODE

Autoimmune hepatitis: K75.4

1. *AIH* is defined as an "unresolving inflammation of the liver of unknown cause" (Manns et al., 2010, p. 1).
2. AIH can progress to cirrhosis and/or hepatocellular carcinoma.
3. Presence of ANA and/or SMA is associated with autoimmune hepatitis.
4. Immunosuppressive medications are usually required to manage AIH.
5. Liver transplantation is an option for those who qualify.

REFERENCES

Czaja, A. J. (2015). Autoimmune hepatitis: Diagnosis. In P. R. McNally (Ed.), *GI/liver secrets plus* (5th ed., pp. 121–132). Philadelphia, PA: Elsevier Saunders.

Lucey, M. R., & Vierling, J. M. (2014). Clinical presentation and natural history of autoimmune hepatitis. *Clinical Liver Disease, 3*(1), 9–11.

Manns, M. P., Czaja, A. J., Gorham, J. D., Krawitt, E. L., Mieli-Vergani, G., Vergani, D., & Vierling, J. M. (2010). Diagnosis and management of autoimmune hepatitis. *Hepatology, 51*(6), 2193–2213.

Manns, M. P., & Taubert, R. (2014). Treatment of autoimmune hepatitis. *Clinical Liver Disease, 3*(1), 15–17.

20

Acute Liver Failure

Acute liver failure (ALF) is a condition in which there is severe liver dysfunction with hepatic encephalopathy and compromised liver function (identified as severe coagulopathy; Goldberg & Chopra, 2016). Symptoms usually progress over a period of 1 to 2 weeks (Fix, 2013). ALF can occur for a variety of reasons (Table 20.1) The patient with ALF usually does not have a preexisting liver condition or cirrhosis. Less than half of patients with ALF will naturally recover. When recognized, patients should be referred to a transplant center for urgent evaluation and treatment (Goldberg & Chopra, 2016).

At the end of this chapter, the reader will be able to:

1. Define ALF
2. Identify two prophylactic approaches that are important to minimize risk of complications in the patient with ALF
3. Discuss treatment strategies for the patient with ALF

TABLE 20.1 Reasons for ALF

Acetaminophen toxicity

Acute fatty liver of pregnancy

Acute hepatitis A or B infection

Autoimmune hepatitis

Budd–Chiari syndrome

Herpes simplex virus infection

Mushroom poisoning

Wilson's disease

Unknown

ALF, acute liver failure.
Source: Goldberg and Chopra (2016).

CONCERNS FOR THE PATIENT WITH ACUTE LIVER FAILURE

The patient with ALF has a high risk of mortality. Complications that can arise include hemodynamic instability and infection (commonly of the blood, urinary tract, or respiratory tract). These patients have a degree of hepatic encephalopathy and coagulopathy with highly elevated transaminases (Goldberg & Chopra, 2016). Multisystem organ failure (MSOF) can develop, including respiratory and renal failure. Other complications can include cerebral edema and infection (Fix, 2013).

PERTINENT LABORTORY FINDINGS

Laboratory testing that is performed includes serial liver profiles (particularly aspartate aminotransferase [AST] and alanine transaminase [ALT] levels), bilirubin levels, coagulation factors (international normalized ratio [INR]), complete blood count, and complete metabolic panel to check for electrolyte imbalances and renal failure. These patients frequently develop hypoglycemia, hypomagnesemia, hypocalcemia, and hypophosphatemia (Goldberg & Chopra, 2016).

ALF can occur rapidly and without warning. These patients may become unstable quickly because of low systemic vascular resistance that is associated with ALF. Fluid resuscitation is a priority and must be given cautiously, as fluid overload can cause cerebral edema. The goal for the mean arterial pressure (MAP) is 75 mmHg to maintain adequate perfusion to vital organs. Vasopressors may be required, including norepinephrine and vasopressin (Goldberg & Chopra, 2016).

If ALF is related to acetaminophen toxicity, N-acetylcysteine (NAC) is given intravenously (Goldberg & Chopra, 2016). NAC infusion may also be of benefit for patients with other etiologies of liver disease with lower grades of hepatic encephalopathy (Fix, 2013).

There are several prevention strategies that are a part of managing the patient with ALF. Coagulopathy is common in patients with ALF, sometimes with an INR in the 7 to 10 range. In order to decrease bleeding risk, blood products may need to be given. It is not recommended that fresh frozen plasma be given for prophylaxis. Patients should be on stress ulcer prophylaxis with a proton pump inhibitor to minimize risk of gastrointestinal (GI) bleeding. All patients with ALF should have routine chest radiographs, and blood, urine, and sputum cultures. If ascites is present, diagnostic paracentesis should be performed to rule out spontaneous bacterial peritonitis. Prophylactic antibiotics are not recommended unless clinical deterioration is present. During this process, metabolic rates are increased and nutrition is hugely important. Enteral feedings may be needed if the patient is unable to meet his or her nutritional requirements. Metabolic imbalances are common, including acid–base imbalance, hypomagnesemia, hyponatremia, hypokalemia, hypophosphatemia, and hypoglycemia. Hepatic encephalopathy (HE) exists with ALF, and is thought to be related to increased ammonia levels in the bloodstream. HE should be managed aggressively; prevention of HE progression to coma is ideal. Lactulose is commonly used to bind to ammonia and is removed through the gut. Worsened states of HE (grade 3 or 4) have been associated with cerebral edema and seizures caused by increased intracranial pressure (ICP) and usually requires endotracheal intubation for airway protection (Goldberg & Chopra, 2016; Lee, Larson, & Stravitz, 2012). Ways of preventing increased ICP include elevating the head of the bed; promoting an even fluid balance; reducing agitation and stimulation; providing a calm, soothing environment; and hypertonic saline administration. The goal of cerebral perfusion pressure (CPP) is 60 to 80 mmHg (Goldberg & Chopra, 2016; Lee et al., 2012). Acute renal failure (ARF) develops in approximately 40% of patients with ALF, and is associated with higher mortality. Continuous renal replacement therapy may be needed to maintain fluid balance and stabilize the patient's hemodynamics. In approximately 30% of patients, pulmonary infections or edema can occur (Goldberg & Chopra, 2016).

Twenty-five percent of patients with ALF will receive a liver transplant. Survival rates after 1 year are approximately 84% (Fix, 2013).

ICD-10 CODE

Liver disease, unspecified: K 76.9
Toxic liver disease with acute hepatitis: K71.2
HELLP [hemolysis, elevated liver enzymes, low platelet count] syndrome, unspecified trimester: O14.20

FAST FACTS in a NUTSHELL

1. ALF is a condition in which there is severe liver dysfunction with hepatic encephalopathy and compromised liver function (identified as severe coagulopathy).
2. The patient with ALF should be sent to a transplant center for urgent liver transplant evaluation.
3. A key to survival for the patient with ALF is to prevent infection and MSOF.
4. ALF can cause many severe complications, even death. Prompt recognition and proper referral to an expert are essential for survival.

REFERENCES

Fix, O. K. (2013). Acute liver failure: Peritransplant management and outcomes. *Clinical Liver Disease, 2*(4), 165–168.

Goldberg, E., & Chopra, S. (2016). Acute liver failure in adults: Management and prognosis. Retrieved from www.uptodate.com/contents/acute-liver-failure-in-adults-management-and-prognosis?source=search_result&search=Acute+liver+failure+in+adults&selectedTitle=2%7E150.html

Lee, W. M., Larson, A. M., & Stravitz, R. T. (2012). AASLD position paper: The management of acute liver failure: Update 2011. *Hepatology, 55*(3), 676–684.

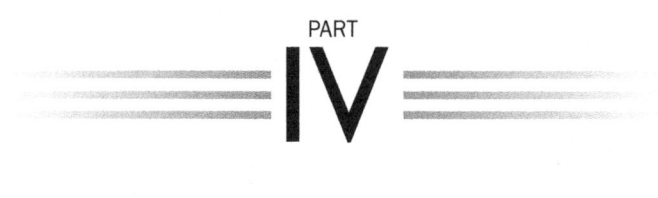

PART

IV

Cirrhosis and Its Complications

21

Cirrhosis

*Cirrhosis, also known as end-stage liver disease, is the fi-
nal stage of liver fibrosis progression. The cirrhotic liver is
distorted at the cellular level and regenerative nodules are
present from repeated liver injury over years (Goldberg &
Chopra, 2015). It is the twelfth leading cause of death in
the United States, responsible for approximately 40,000
deaths per year (Kumar, Abbas, & Aster, 2014; Murray et al.,
2013). The U.S. health care costs associated with cirrhosis
are approximately $4 billion per year as the disease affects
over 2 million people (Kanwal & El-Serag, 2013). Cirrhosis
can develop for a variety of reasons (Figure 21.1), with
the most common causes being alcohol consumption, viral
hepatitis, and nonalcoholic steatohepatitis. Complications
of cirrhosis can be fatal. Management goals are to prevent
complications and to preserve quality of life.*

At the end of this book, the reader will be able to:

1. State three of the most common causes of cirrhosis
2. Name four possible complications of cirrhosis
3. Discuss treatment strategies for managing cirrhosis

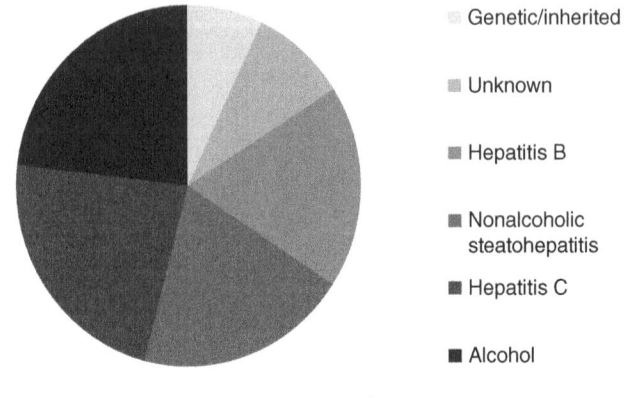

FIGURE 21.1 Common causes of cirrhosis.

COMPLICATIONS OF CIRRHOSIS

Cirrhosis is divided into two subsets: compensated and de-compensated. *Compensated cirrhosis* is defined as the absence of any of the complications of cirrhosis with the liver maintaining adequate function at the cellular level. On the other hand, *decompensated cirrhosis* develops when one or more complications of cirrhosis have occurred. There is an increased morbidity and mortality when complications of cirrhosis occur. Complications of cirrhosis include:

- Ascites
- Spontaneous bacterial peritonitis
- Hepatic encephalopathy
- Hepatorenal syndrome
- Hepatopulmonary syndrome
- Hepatocellular carcinoma
- Variceal hemorrhage

Once these complications have developed, patients should be referred to a transplant center for evaluation for liver transplant (Goldberg & Chopra, 2015). Patients with cirrhosis are at a higher risk for developing infections. Prophylactic antibiotics are recommended for certain patients with cirrhosis (Fernandez & Arroyo, 2013).

ASSESSMENT FINDINGS

There are many nonspecific symptoms that can be associated with cirrhosis, including fatigue, weakness, loss of appetite, and weight loss. Patients may notice they bruise more easily; women may experience amenorrhea or irregular menstrual cycles; men may experience impotence and loss of sex drive. Patients will also experience confusion (noticed by caregivers), itching and/ or yellowing of skin or whites of eyes, abdominal distension or bloating, or lower extremity edema. Patients may have signs of anemia and should be questioned as to whether they have bloody or black stools (Goldberg & Chopra, 2015).

Physical examination findings may include jaundice (skin and scleral icterus), low systemic blood pressure, signs of portal hypertension (ascites, melena, hematochezia, or hematemesis), hepatomegaly, splenomegaly, caput medusa (bulging veins along abdominal wall), confusion, asterixis, spider angiomatas, gynecomastia, lower extremity pitting edema, Dupuytren's contracture, palmer erythema, severe muscle cramps, and clubbing/nail changes (Goldberg & Chopra, 2015).

PERTINENT LABORATORY FINDINGS

Patients with cirrhosis may have abnormal liver function test (LFT) readings, hyperbilirubinemia, elevated international normalized ratio (INR), thrombocytopenia, anemia, leukopenia, hyponatremia, hypoalbuminemia, renal insufficiency, and glucose intolerance (Goldberg & Chopra, 2015).

IMAGING STUDIES

Occasionally, cirrhosis is an incidental finding on imaging studies, such as ultrasound, CT scan, or MRI. If cirrhosis is assumed, ultrasound is performed to investigate the liver tissue and determine vascular flow. Common terms used if cirrhosis is present on imaging studies include *asymmetrical, uneven texture, nodular,* and *contracted* or *small*. The gold standard for determining the presence and staging of cirrhosis is a liver biopsy (Goldberg & Chopra, 2015).

PROGNOSIS MODELS

The Child–Turcott-Pugh score was created in the 1960s to estimate the severity of cirrhosis. It is a calculation based on total bilirubin, INR, and albumin levels, and takes into account the presence of ascites and encephalopathy. Results are calculated in the range of 5 to 15, and placed in categories of A, B, or C and provide an estimation of mortality (Cholongitas et al., 2005). This score was used to prioritize the waiting list for liver transplants from 1997 until 2002 (Kalra, Wedd, & Biggins, 2016).

The Model for End-Stage Liver Disease (MELD) score was developed by Russell H. Wiesner in 2001. This score takes into account the total bilirubin, INR, and creatinine levels, as well as whether a patient has developed renal failure that requires dialysis. The MELD is used by the United Network for Organ Sharing (UNOS) to prioritize the waiting list for liver transplant, placing the most urgent need at the top of the list. The scores range from 9 to 40, with less than 9 signifying it is too early for transplant and 40 indicating an urgent need for transplant. This scoring system estimates 3-month mortality in patients with chronic liver disease (Wiesner et al., 2003).

Because hyponatremia has been shown to affect mortality in patients with cirrhosis (Kim et al., 2008), the UNOS approved a policy to include serum sodium levels as a part of the MELD score calculation. As of January 2016, the new MELD-Na score is used to prioritize the waiting list for liver transplantation if the patient's MELD is greater than 11 (Kalra et al., 2016).

TABLE 21.1 Child–Turcott–Pugh Scores

Score	1-Year Survival (%)	2-Year Survival (%)
A (5–6)	~100	85
B (7–9)	81	57
C (10–15)	45	35

TABLE 21.2 MELD Scoring

Score	3-Month Mortality (%)
40 or more	71.3
30–39	52.6
2029	19.6
10–19	6
< 9	1.9

MELD, Model for End-Stage Liver Disease.

MANAGEMENT

The goals of therapy for the patient with cirrhosis include slowing the development of cirrhosis, preserving liver function as long as possible, reducing the possibility of further injury, preventing complications of cirrhosis, recognizing and promptly treating the complications of cirrhosis, and recognizing appropriate time for liver transplantation evaluation (Goldberg & Chopra, 2015). Patients with cirrhosis should undergo screening measures to avoid complications, including regular esophagogastroduodenoscopy (EGD) to appropriately manage varices and prevent bleeding episodes, and imaging studies to rule out hepatocellular carcinoma. Patients with cirrhosis should have vaccinations for hepatitis A and B, if they not already done so. Also, regular influenza and pneumococcal immunizations, as well as diphtheria and tetanus boosters are recommended per standard protocols. Optimal nutrition is essential to maintain ideal health for patients with cirrhosis (Yadav & Vargas, 2015). Specific complications of cirrhosis are discussed in subsequent chapters.

ICD-10 CODE

Unspecified cirrhosis of liver: K74.60
Other cirrhosis of liver: K74.69
Toxic liver disease with fibrosis and cirrhosis of the liver: K71.7

1. The most common causes of cirrhosis are viral hepatitis, nonalcoholic steatohepatitis, and alcohol consumption.
2. Complications of cirrhosis can be fatal; referral for liver transplantation is recommended.
3. Treatment strategies are aimed at slowing the development of cirrhosis, preserving liver function as long as possible, reducing the possibility of further liver injury, preventing complications of cirrhosis, recognizing and promptly treating complications of cirrhosis, and recognizing the appropriate time for liver transplantation evaluation.

REFERENCES

Cholongitas, E., Papatheodoridis, G. V., Vangeli, M., Terreni, N., Patch, D., & Burroughs, A. K. (2005). Systematic review: The model for end-stage liver disease—Should it replace Child-Pugh's classification for assessing prognosis in cirrhosis? *Alimentary Pharmacology & Therapeutics, 22*(11–12), 1079–89. doi:10.1111/j.1365-2036.2005.02691.x

Fernandez, J., & Arroyo, V. (2013). Bacterial infections in cirrhosis: A growing problem with significant implications. *Clinical Liver Disease, 2*(3), 102–105.

Goldberg, E., & Chopra, S. (2015). Cirrhosis in adults: Overview of complications, general management, and prognosis & Cirrhosis in adults: Etiologies, clinical manifestations, and diagnosis. Retrieved from www.uptodate.com/contents/cirrhosis-in-adults-overview-of-complications-general-management-and-prognosis?source=search_re sult&search=Cirrhosis+in+adults%3A+Overview&selectedTitle =1%7E150.html

Kalra, A., Wedd, J. P., & Biggins, S. W. (2016). Changing prioritization for transplantation: MELD-Na, hepatocellular carcinoma exceptions, and more. *Current Opinion in Organ Transplantation, 21,*120–126.

Kanwal, F., & El-Serag, H. (2013). Improving quality of care in patients with cirrhosis. *Clinical Liver Disease, 2*(3), 123–124.

Kim, W. R., Biggins, S. W., Kremers, W. K., Wiesner, R. H., Kamath, P. S., Benson, J. T., . . . Therneau, T. M. (2008). Hyponatremia and mortality among patients on the liver transplant waiting list. *New England Journal of Medicine, 359 (10),* 1018–1026.

Kumar, V., Abbas, A., & Aster, J. C. (2014). *Robbins & Cotran: Pathologic basis of disease* (9th ed.). St. Louis, MO: Elsevier.

Murray, C. J., Atkinson, C., Bhalla, K., Birbeck, G., Burstein, R., Chou, D., . . . U.S. Burden of Disease Collaborators. (2013). The state of US health, 1990–2010: burden of disease, injuries, and risk factors. *JAMA, 310*(6), 591–608.

Wiesner, R., Edwards, E., Freeman, R., Harper, A., Kim, R., Kamath, P., . . . United Network for Organ Sharing Liver Disease Severity Score Committee. (2003). Model for end-stage liver disease (MELD) and allocation of donor livers. *Gastroenterology, 124*(1), 91–96.

Yadav, A., & Vargas, H. E. (2015). Care of the patient with cirrhosis. *Clinical Liver Disease, 5*(4), 100–104.

22

Ascites/Fluid Retention

One of the most common complications of cirrhosis is ascites, or the accumulation of fluid in the abdominal cavity. Ascites that develops from cirrhosis is associated with portal hypertension. As the liver becomes damaged and cirrhotic, it becomes difficult for blood to flow through the liver cells (sinusoids). This causes splanchnic vasodilation by release of vasodilators (e.g., nitric oxide) into the bloodstream. The body reacts by stimulating the sympathetic nervous system, the renin–angiotensin–aldosterone pathway, and the antidiuretic hormone, causing increased levels of vasopressin, angiotensin, and aldosterone thereby producing renal vasoconstriction and increased sodium and water absorption. The increased pressure in the capillaries and changes in osmotic pressure allow fluid to move from the bloodstream into the peritoneal cavity (i.e., ascites; Chaney, 2015; Runyon, 2013; Yadav & Vargas, 2015). This chapter discusses ascites and appropriate treatment strategies.

At the end of this chapter, the reader will be able to:

1. Name two physical examination findings that the patient with cirrhosis and ascites may have
2. State why a diagnostic paracentesis would be needed for a patient with ascites and cirrhosis
3. Describe the treatment goal for the patient with ascites and cirrhosis

ASSESSMENT FINDINGS

The patient with cirrhosis and ascites may complain of increased weight gain, lower extremity edema, and abdominal bloating or distension. Physical examination findings may reveal a distended or even tense abdomen, positive fluid wave, dullness to abdominal percussion, and peripheral edema. The patient may be hypotensive.

PERTINENT LABORATORY FINDINGS

A diagnostic paracentesis is recommended. Ascites fluid should be sent for total protein and albumin level tests, cell count with differential, and bacterial cultures. A serum–ascites–albumin gradient (SAAG) is calculated, with a number greater than or equal to 1.1 g/dL diagnostic of ascites from portal hypertension (Yadav & Vargas, 2015). Routine laboratory testing, such as complete blood count, complete metabolic panel, and liver function testing, should be performed with new-onset ascites and at routine return visits. Patients with cirrhosis and ascites can develop electrolyte imbalances and renal failure, so close monitoring is essential.

IMAGING STUDIES

Ultrasound is helpful to determine whether ascites is present if there is any uncertainty upon physical examination. CT and MRI will identify ascites as well, but are not recommended for identification-purposes only. These studies may be necessary for other reasons.

DIFFERENTIAL DIAGNOSIS

Patients may develop ascites for reasons other than cirrhosis. These include:

- Acute liver failure
- Alcoholic hepatitis
- Budd–Chiari syndrome
- Heart failure
- Malignancies (e.g., hepatocellular carcinoma)
- Nephrotic syndrome
- Pancreatitis
- Sinusoidal obstruction syndrome

MANAGEMENT

Once ascites develops as a complication of cirrhosis, 85% of those affected survive after 1 year, and 44% of patients survive after 5 years. If ascites is identified, a diagnostic paracentesis is recommended. A SAAG should be calculated to verify portal hypertension as a cause of ascites. If the patient with cirrhosis is hospitalized, it is recommended that a diagnostic paracentesis be performed to rule out spontaneous bacterial peritonitis (Yadav & Vargas, 2015).

Patient education is essential to prevent further decompensation. Patients should abstain from all alcohol consumption and avoid using nonsteroidal anti-inflammatory drugs (NSAIDs; can cause further liver and renal injury). Patients should make several dietary changes, including restricting sodium intake to less than 2 g per day. Fluid restriction may be needed if serum sodium levels become low (less than 125 mmol/L). Diuretics (furosemide [40 mg daily] and spironolactone [100 mg daily]) are the mainstay treatment. Electrolytes, particularly potassium and sodium, should be monitored closely. If renal function declines and severe hyponatremia or worsened hepatic encephalopathy develop, diuretics should be stopped. If the patient has been previously treated for hypertension with angiotensin-converting enzyme (ACE) inhibitors or angiotensin receptor blockers (ARBs), these medications should be discontinued as lower blood pressure can cause renal injury and increase mortality. Ascites can become infected, called *spontaneous bacterial peritonitis* (SBP). Patients with low-protein ascites (ascitic protein less than 1.5 g/dL) and renal impairment or patients with liver failure can have a higher incidence of developing SBP. Prophylaxis is recommended in these cases with norfloxacin (not available in the United States) or trimethoprim/sulfamethoxazole (Bactrim; Runyon, 2013).

If diuretics are not tolerated and diet changes do not improve fluid accumulation (refractory ascites), patients may need serial therapeutic paracentesis for symptom relief. Some patients may need this as often as twice a week if fluid accumulates quickly. Intravenous albumin should be given for fluid replacement, as large volumes can be removed at one time (up to 10 to 15 L). Midodrine has been associated with better clinical outcomes in the patient with refractory ascites. This is thought to be related to increasing blood pressure (which is normally low in this patient population) and renal perfusion. Doses of 7.5 mg three times per day are recommended in certain cases. A procedure called *transjugular intrahepatic portosystemic stent-shunt* (TIPS) may be recommended to divert blood flow from the liver (portal vein) to one of the hepatic veins, thereby bypassing the liver and reducing portal hypertension and the complications of ascites and gastrointestinal bleeding (varices). All patients with cirrhosis and ascites should be evaluated for liver transplantation at a transplant center (Runyon, 2013).

ICD-10 CODE

Other ascites: R18.8
Toxic liver disease with chronic active hepatitis with ascites: K71.51
Edema, unspecified (fluid retention): R60.9

1. Patients with ascites may have symptoms, including increased abdominal distension, weight gain, hypotension, and peripheral edema.
2. Antihypertensive medications (ACE/ARB) should be discontinued as lower blood pressure can cause renal injury and increase mortality.
3. The first-line treatment for patients with cirrhosis and ascites is dietary modification (sodium restriction) and diuretic therapy.
4. Ascites can become infected, called *spontaneous bacterial peritonitis* (SBP), and patients with low-protein ascites (ascitic protein less than 1.5 g/dL) and renal impairment or patients with liver failure can have a higher incidence of developing SBP. Prophylaxis is recommended in these cases.
5. A procedure called *transjugular intrahepatic portosystemic stent-shunt* (TIPS) may be recommended for patients with refractory ascites.

REFERENCES

Chaney, A. (2015). Cirrhosis complications: Ascites and spontaneous bacterial peritonitis. *Clinician Reviews, 25*(4), 33–37.

Runyon, B. (2013). Introduction to the revised American Association for the Study of Liver Diseases practice guideline. Management of adult patients with ascites due to cirrhosis: Update 2012. *Hepatology, 57*(4), 1651–1653.

Yadav, A., & Vargas, H. E. (2015). Care of the patient with cirrhosis. *Clinical Liver Disease, 5*(4), 100–104.

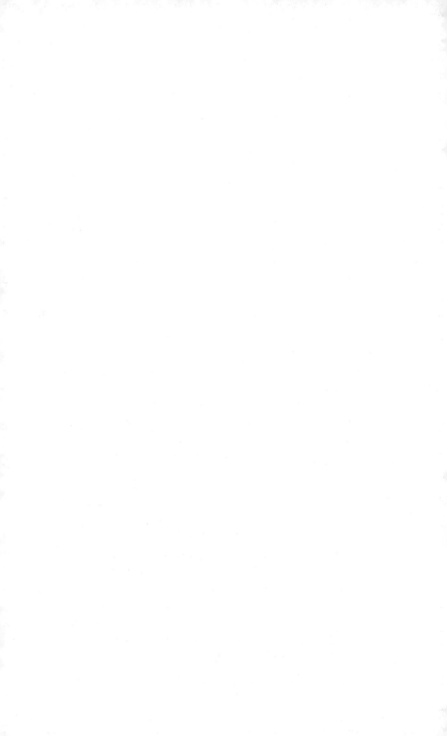

23

Spontaneous Bacterial Peritonitis

Spontaneous bacterial peritonitis (SBP) is a complication of cirrhosis that can develop in patients with cirrhosis and ascites, occurring in approximately 25% of these patients. Translocation of bacteria (most commonly Escherichia coli, Klebsiella pneumoniae, *and* Streptococcus pneumonia) *from the intestine into the bloodstream and ascites is commonly blamed. Diagnosis is made when the ascitic fluid (obtained by diagnostic paracentesis) shows an absolute polymorphonuclear (PMN) leukocyte count greater than or equal to 250 cells/mm^3 and/or positive ascitic fluid cultures. When there is only an elevated PMN cell count with negative cultures, this is termed* neutrocytic ascites *(treated the same as SBP). There are certain risk factors associated with the development of SBP, including gastrointestinal bleeding, prior SBP episodes, and low ascitic total protein levels. SBP is associated with a higher mortality, especially if left untreated, it may lead to sepsis and septic shock with multisystem organ failure (Chaney, 2015; Runyon, 2013; Yadav & Vargas, 2015).*

At the end of this chapter, the reader will be able to:

1. Define how spontaneous bacterial peritonitis is diagnosed
2. Name four signs and symptoms of SBP
3. Discuss treatment strategies for SBP

ASSESSMENT FINDINGS

Some patients with SBP may be asymptomatic. Others may present with fever (temperature greater than 100°F), chills, abdominal pain or tenderness, altered mental status or confusion (worsened hepatic encephalopathy), presence of systemic inflammatory response syndrome (SIRS) criteria (see Table 23.1), nausea, vomiting, constipation, or diarrhea (Chaney, 2015; Goldberg & Chopra, 2015). Some patients develop a small bowel obstruction, or ileus, at the time of SBP infection.

PERTINENT LABORATORY FINDINGS

Diagnostic paracentesis should be performed when there is a suspicion of SBP. Fluid should be sent for tests of cell count with differential, albumin, total protein, Gram stain, bacterial aerobic and anaerobic cultures, glucose, lactate dehydrogenase, and amylase (Runyon, 2013).

Other laboratory testing should include complete blood count, complete metabolic panel, and liver function testing. Acidosis and/or leukocytosis can be associated with SBP and should be noted. Blood and urine cultures may be required to evaluate for sepsis. Renal failure can occur with SBP episodes and is associated with a higher mortality rate. Careful monitoring of the patient's renal function is essential.

TABLE 23.1 Systemic Inflammatory Response Syndrome (SIRS) Criteria

Finding	Abnormality
Temperature	> 100.4°F or < 96.8°F
Heart rate	> 90 beats/min
Respiratory findings	> 20 breaths/min or arterial carbon dioxide ($PaCO_2$) <32 mmHg
White cell count	> 12,000/μL or < 4,000/μL or > 10% immature neutrophils (band forms)

Presence of two or more criteria diagnostic for SIRS.

Ultrasound is usually performed at the time of diagnostic paracentesis to ensure that an adequate fluid pocket is available for sampling. Other imaging studies, such as CT or MRI scan, may be indicated if another source of infection is considered to be the cause of development of SBP (bowel perforation, recent intra-abdominal surgery, pancreatitis, etc.).

MANAGEMENT

Patients with neutrocytic ascites or SBP should be treated with broad-spectrum antibiotics. Administration of cefotaxime 2 g intravenously every 8 hours (or ceftriaxone 2 g every 24 hours) for 7 days has been proven effective in treating most SBP cases. Patients should be given intravenous albumin on the day of diagnosis (1.5 g/kg) and again on hospital day 3 (1 g/kg) to prevent renal deterioration and to reduce mortality. Some providers perform a repeat paracentesis after 2 to 3 days of antibiotics to ensure improvement in infection and response to treatment (decrease in ascitic fluid cell count; Runyon, 2013; Yadav & Vargas, 2015).

There has been some association with SBP and proton pump inhibitor (PPI) use. If a PPI is not needed for active treatment of a gastrointestinal issue, it is recommended that this medication be stopped. Patients who have had an episode of SBP should complete the treatment course of antibiotics and then start prophylactic antibiotics for prevention of further episodes. Norfloxacin (not available in the United States) or trimethoprim/sulfamethoxazole (Bactrim) is recommended for daily dosing for SBP prevention (Runyon, 2013).

ICD-10 CODE

Spontaneous bacterial peritonitis: K65.2
Peritonitis, unspecified: K65.9
Generalized acute peritonitis: K65.0

1. The most common causes of SBP are *E. coli*, *K. pneumoniae*, and *S. pneumonia*.
2. SBP diagnosis is made when the ascitic fluid (obtained by diagnostic paracentesis) shows an absolute PMN leukocyte count greater than or equal to 250 cells/mm^3 and/or positive ascitic fluid cultures.
3. Neutrocytic ascites occurs when there is only an elevated PMN cell count with negative cultures.
4. Risk factors associated with the development of SBP include gastrointestinal bleeding, prior SBP episodes, and low ascitic total protein levels.
5. Patients with SBP may have fever (temperature greater than 100°F), chills, abdominal pain or tenderness, altered mental status or confusion (worsened hepatic encephalopathy), presence of systemic inflammatory response syndrome (SIRS) criteria, nausea, vomiting, and constipation or diarrhea.
6. Diagnostic paracentesis should be performed when there is a suspicion of SBP.
7. SBP treatment includes cefotaxime 2 g intravenously every 8 hours (or ceftriaxone 2 gm every 24 hours) for 7 days, followed by either norfloxacin or trimethoprim/sulfamethoxazole (Bactrim) for prevention of future episodes.
8. Patients should be given intravenous albumin on the day of diagnosis (1.5 g/kg) and again on hospital day 3 (1 g/kg) to prevent renal deterioration and to reduce mortality.

REFERENCES

Chaney, A. (2015). Cirrhosis complications: Ascites and spontaneous bacterial peritonitis. *Clinician Reviews, 25*(4), 33–37.

Goldberg, E., & Chopra, S. (2015). Cirrhosis in adults: Overview of complications, general management, and prognosis & cirrhosis in adults: Etiologies, clinical manifestations, and diagnosis. Retrieved from www.uptodate.com/contents/cirrhosis-in-adults-overview-of-complications-general-management-and-prognosis?source=search_result&search=Cirrhosis+in+adults%3A+Overview&selectedTitle=1%7E150.html

Runyon, B. (2013). Introduction to the revised American Association for the Study of Liver Diseases practice guideline. Management of adult patients with ascites due to cirrhosis: Update 2012. *Hepatology, 57*(4), 1651–1653.

Yadav, A., & Vargas, H. E. (2015). Care of the patient with cirrhosis. *Clinical Liver Disease, 5*(4), 100–104.

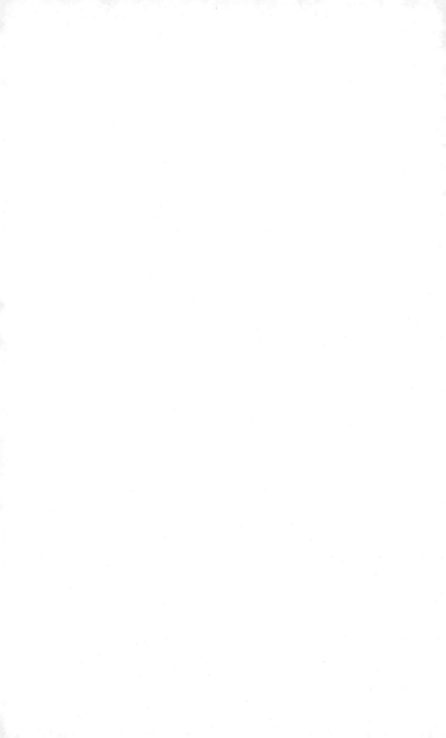

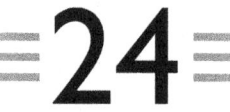

24

Gastrointestinal Bleeding

Another development that can occur from portal hypertension is gastroesophageal varices. Approximately 50% of patients with cirrhosis will develop varices. Risk factors for variceal hemorrhage or bleeding include advanced cirrhosis, increased size of varices, and presence of red wale signs seen on esophagogastroduodenoscopy (EGD; Garcia-Tsao et al., 2009; Yadav & Vargas, 2015). Complications of variceal hemorrhage can include infection, severe anemia, and death. It is important to prevent variceal hemorrhage, and, if hemorrhage does occur to manage promptly.

At the end of this chapter, the reader will be able to:

1. Discuss the signs and symptoms of esophageal varices and variceal hemorrhage
2. Name two medications used to manage variceal hemorrhage
3. State when repeat EGDs should be performed after an episode of variceal hemorrhage

ASSESSMENT FINDINGS

Providers should note patient history of melena, hematemesis, hematochezia, syncope, dizziness, palpitations, or prior history of gastrointestinal (GI) bleeding. Physical examination may reveal abdominal pain or tenderness, tachycardia, hypotension, orthostatic hypotension, and bloody or black stool on rectal examination. Signs of cirrhosis may be present (see Chapter 21).

PERTINENT LABORATORY FINDINGS

Routine laboratory testing, such as complete blood count, complete metabolic panel, prothrombin/international normalized ratio (PT/INR), and liver function testing, should be performed on all patients suspected of having variceal hemorrhage. Patients may require serial hemoglobin and hematocrit (H&H) to check for worsening anemia. An updated type and cross-match are recommended in case blood transfusions are required. Coagulopathy may be present, and correction will be necessary if active bleeding is present.

DIAGNOSTIC STUDIES/MANAGEMENT

EGD is the gold standard when it comes to diagnosing gastroesophageal varices. When a diagnosis of cirrhosis is made, it is recommended that an EGD be performed to screen for varices. If noted, varices should be graded as small or large. Presence of red wale signs on EGD should be documented, as this is a risk factor for developing variceal hemorrhage. If no varices are present on EGD screening, then repeat EGD should be done in 3 years. If patient develops issues with decompensation of liver disease or signs of variceal hemorrhage are present, EGD should be performed at that time and then annually thereafter. If small varices are present and beta blockers are not prescribed, repeat EGD should be done after 2 years. If moderate to large varices are present and the patient is at high risk for variceal hemorrhage, EGD with endoscopic variceal ligation (EVL) can be performed and/or starting the patient on a beta blocker is recommended (Garcia-Tsao et al., 2009).

Within 24 hours of a variceal hemorrhage, an EGD should be done following adequate stabilization of hemodynamics. If the patient remains unstable despite fluid resuscitation and blood transfusions, EGD should be done within 12 hours. At the time of the procedure, EVL and sclerotherapy are approaches used to control bleeding (Sandhu & Strate, 2015).

Prevention of variceal hemorrhage is key for variceal management. Use of nonselective beta blockers (NSBB), such as carvedilol, nadolol, and propranolol, are recommended for patients at high risk for hemorrhage. For patients who cannot tolerate an NSBB, EVL is an option (Garcia-Tsao et al., 2009; Yadav & Vargas, 2015).

Patients with variceal hemorrhage require urgent hospital admission to the intensive care unit (ICU). Central line and/or large-bore intravenous access is necessary (Sandhu & Strate, 2015). Latest treatment guidelines recommend that goal hemoglobin be targeted around 7 g/dL for optimal mortality benefit. Patients who have developed variceal hemorrhage are at a higher risk for developing infection. Antibiotics should be given as a preventative measure, with ceftriaxone for 5 to 7 days as the antibiotic of choice. In addition, intravenous octreotide is given as a continuous infusion for 3 to 5 days to cause splanchnic vasoconstriction, which can reduce bleeding. In some patients, a transjugular intrahepatic portosystemic stent-shunt (TIPS) procedure can be used to control and prevent future episodes of variceal hemorrhage. Patients with varices who have had an episode of variceal hemorrhage should be considered for liver transplantation (Garcia-Tsao et al., 2009; Runyon, 2013).

ICD-10 CODE

Gastric varices: I86.4
Esophageal varices without bleeding: I85.00
Esophageal varices with bleeding: I85.01
Gastrointestinal hemorrhage, unspecified: K92.2

1. Gastroesophageal varices occur in approximately 50% of patients with cirrhosis.
2. Risk factors for variceal hemorrhage or bleeding include advanced cirrhosis, increased size of varices, and presence of red wale signs seen on EGD.
3. Complications of variceal hemorrhage can include infection, severe anemia, and death.
4. It is important to prevent variceal hemorrhage, and, if hemorrhage does occur, to manage promptly.
5. EGD is the gold standard used to diagnose gastroesophageal varices.
6. Options for managing varices include nonselective beta blockers and esophageal variceal ligation by EGD.

REFERENCES

Garcia-Tsao, G., Sanyal, A. J., Grace, N. D., Carey, W., the Practice Guidelines Committee of the American Association for the Study of Liver Diseases, & the Practice Parameters Committee of the American College of Gastroenterology. (2009). Prevention and management of gastroesophagealvarices and variceal hemorrhage in cirrhosis. *Hepatology, 46*(3), 922–938.

Runyon, B. (2013). Introduction to the revised American Association for the Study of Liver Diseases practice guideline. Management of adult patients with ascites due to cirrhosis: Update 2012. *Hepatology, 57*(4), 1651–1653.

Sandhu, D., & Strate, L. (2015). Upper gastrointestinal hemorrhage. In P. R. McNally (Ed.), *GI/liver secrets plus* (5th ed., pp. 377–383). Philadelphia, PA: Elsevier Saunders.

Yadav, A., & Vargas, H. E. (2015). Care of the patient with cirrhosis. *Clinical Liver Disease, 5*(4), 100–104.

25

Hepatic Encephalopathy

Hepatic encephalopathy (HE) is a neuropsychiatric complication of advanced liver disease that affects both motor and sensory functions of the brain. Symptoms range from mild impairment to a comatose state. Approximately 11% of patients have overt encephalopathy at the time of cirrhosis diagnosis, whereas 22% to 74% of patients have minimal/covert HE (Dhiman, 2015; Yadav & Vargas, 2015). Usually, patients develop HE following a trigger or precipitant. This could be caused by infection, overdiuresis with electrolyte imbalances, medications (sedating), gastrointestinal bleeding, or lack of compliance with HE medications. Classification of HE is divided into grades 1 through 4, and more broadly into covert HE and overt HE. Minimal, or covert HE, is difficult to recognize for many providers, but accurate diagnosis has been associated with better quality of life, decreased risk of accidents, and decreased progression to overt HE (Yadav & Vargas, 2015).

At the end of this chapter, the reader will be able to:

1. Identify the two types of HE
2. Name four findings associated with HE that pertain to patient history or physical examination
3. State three treatment options for managing HE

ASSESSMENT FINDINGS

A thorough history should be performed when evaluating the patient for HE. A sleep disturbance is reported in some patients early in HE development. Caregivers are extremely important in this part of the examination, as patients with HE may be able to "hide" memory loss or mild confusion. Caregivers can verify information given and present an accurate timeline of events to gain a clear picture. History may reveal complaints of mood changes, irritability, excessive sleepiness or fatigue, agitation, poor attention to details, or frequent falls (Dhiman, 2015; Vilstrup et al., 2014).

Physical examination findings include confusion; hyperactive deep tendon reflexes; muscular rigidity; asterixis; and, in cases of severe HE, transient decerebrate posturing and positive Babinski sign (Goldberg & Chopra, 2015; Vilstrup et al., 2014).

DIAGNOSTIC CRITERIA

Covert HE can be very difficult to recognize. When attempting to diagnose covert HE, it is particularly helpful to perform psychometric and neurophysiological tests. This testing should be performed by a psychiatrist or other specialist with experience in evaluating patients with HE (Vilstrup et al., 2014). Covert HE includes West Haven criteria: (a) minimal HE, in which there is no clinical manifestation but there is abnormal psychometric testing, and (b) grade 1 HE, in which the patient is oriented, but symptoms, such as anxiety, irritability, altered sleep habits, or shortened attention span, are evident (Lauridsen & Vilstrup, 2015).

Overt HE can be easier for clinicians to identify. The West Haven criteria (grades 2 through 4) and Glasgow Coma Scale are useful tools to grade the degree of mental impairment. Disorientation and asterixis are common in early stages of overt HE (Dhiman, 2015). In grade 2, the patient is described as confused and lethargic, and may have asterixis on examination. In grade 3, muscular rigidity and hyperreflexia may be present, along with disorientation, strange behavior, delirium, and combativeness. Grade 4 presents as a comatose state (Chaney, Werner, & Kipple, 2015).

PERTINENT LABORATORY FINDINGS

When providers suspect HE in patients with cirrhosis, many times a serum ammonia level is drawn This level may be normal or high in patients with overt HE; therefore, it is highly unreliable to use as a diagnostic tool (Vilstrup et al., 2014).

DIFFERENTIAL DIAGNOSIS

Differential diagnosis for HE can include, but is not limited to:

- Dementia
- Brain lesions
- Obstructive sleep apnea
- Electrolyte disorders
- Stroke or brain hemorrhage
- Organ failure
- Epilepsy
- Drugs (sedating medications such as benzodiazepines, narcotics, and neuroleptics)
- Alcohol
- Complications of diabetes (hyper- or hypoglycemia, ketoacidosis; Vilstrup et al., 2014)

MANAGEMENT

Patients with more severe cases of HE (grades 3 to 4) will require intensive care unit (ICU) admission and, if unable to protect the airway, may need airway protection via intubation and mechanical ventilation. Precipitating factors should be identified and managed appropriately. If infection is considered, a thorough investigation of the cause should be completed and include blood and urine cultures, as well as a diagnostic paracentesis if ascites is present.

There are several medication options for the patients with HE.Lactulose, a nonabsorbable disaccharide, is used as the initial treatment for HE; it is considered an osmotic laxative and patients will have frequent bowel movements while on this medication (Chaney et al., 2015). If the patient is able to tolerate oral intake without concern for aspiration, it is recommended that 20 grams of lactulose be given by mouth every hour until two or three bowel movements have occurred. If the patient's mental state has improved, decreasing the frequency to three to four times per day is appropriate. Most patients maintain controlled HE if they have three to four bowel movements per day. Every patient is different, so medication should be adjusted on an individual basis. Adverse effects of lactulose include diarrhea, perianal skin irritation, dehydration, and hypernatremia. For adherence, patients and caregivers should be well educated on proper use of this medication (Vilstrup et al., 2014).

Rifaximin (Xifaxan) is an antibiotic that is used in the treatment of HE, and to prevent future episodes. The dose is 550 mg twice per day. It is commonly used in conjunction with lactulose (Vilstrup et al., 2014). Adverse effects include abdominal pain, gas, nausea, vomiting, headache, dizziness, and fluid retention. Prior insurance authorization is usually required, which can be frustrating for patients and difficult to obtain (Chaney et al., 2015).

Other medications that can be used in addition or as an alternative to HE medication are oral branched-chain amino acids (BCAAs) and L-ornithine L-aspartate (LOLA; Vilstrup et al., 2014). Options for BCAAs include leucine, isoleucine, and valine (Yadav & Vargas, 2015). Neomycin and metronidazole are also options for treatment of overt HE; however, these have been associated with serious side effects and are not the ideal treatment choice (Vilstrup et al., 2014).

Nutrition plays a large part in HE management. Malnutrition is very common in patients with cirrhosis, occurring in over 75% of cases. Once problems with nutrition occur, they are difficult to manage and it is hard to gain back fat and restore muscle loss. Expert nutrition consultation is recommended for all patients with cirrhosis. Patients should be taught to consume 35 to 40 kcal/kg per day, as well as to *not* restrict protein intake, which should be 1.2 to 1.5 g/kg/day. Small, frequent meals are recommended throughout the day to keep up with nutrition needs (Vilstrup et al., 2014).

ICD-10 CODE

Hepatic failure, with coma: K 72.91
Chronic hepatic failure with coma: K72.11
Hepatic failure, unspecified without coma: K72.90
Chronic hepatic failure without coma: K72.10
Acute and subacute hepatic failure with coma: K72.01
Alcoholic hepatic failure with coma: K70.41
Acute and subacute hepatic failure without coma: K72.00
Alcoholic hepatic failure without coma: K70.40

FAST FACTS in a NUTSHELL

1. Covert (minimal and grade 1) encephalopathy can be difficult to identify.
2. Specialized neuropsychometric testing is necessary for a complete evaluation by an experienced HE clinician.
3. Overt (grades 2 to 4) encephalopathy is easier to recognize than covert HE, and should be aggressively managed to prevent progression of disease.
4. HE is commonly caused by a trigger or precipitant. Efforts to identify the trigger should be prompt and, once identified, treated appropriately.
5. Medication options to treat HE include lactulose, rifaximin, BCAA, and LOLA.
6. Patient and caregiver education about disease, avoiding precipitants, and treatment options is important to prevent reoccurrence of HE and to improve patient survival.
7. Optimal nutrition is important to improve patient outcomes.

REFERENCES

Chaney, A., Werner, K. T., & Kipple, T. (2015). Primary care management of hepatic encephalopathy: A common complication of cirrhosis. *Journal for Nurse Practitioners, 11*(3), 300–306.

Dhiman, R. K. (2015). Impact of minimal/covert hepatic encephalopathy on patients with cirrhosis. *Clinical Liver Disease, 5*(3), 75–78.

Goldberg, E., & Chopra, S. (2015). Cirrhosis in adults: Etiologies, clinical manifestations, and diagnosis. Retrieved from www.uptodate.com/contents/cirrhosis-in-adults-etiologies-clinical-manifestations-and-diagnosis?source=search_result&search=cirrhosis&selectedTitle=1%7E150.html

Lauridsen, M. M., & Vilstrup, H. (2015). Diagnosing covert hepatic encephalopathy. *Clinical Liver Disease, 5*(3), 71–74.

Vilstrup, H., Amodio, P., Bajaj, J., Cordoba, J., Ferenci, P., Mullen, K. D., . . . Wong, P. (2014). Hepatic encephalopathy in chronic liver disease: 2014 practice guideline by AASLD and EASL. *Hepatology, 60*(2), 716–735.

Yadav, A., & Vargas, H. E. (2015). Care of the patient with cirrhosis. *Clinical Liver Disease, 5*(4), 100–104.

26

Hepatorenal Syndrome

Hepatorenal syndrome (HRS) is a condition seen in patients with cirrhosis and ascites in which there is deterioration of the kidneys. This is evidenced by a creatinine level of greater than or equal to 1.5 mg/dL, with no improvement after 2 days of hydration (albumin/volume expanders) and discontinuation of diuretics, no recent use of nephrotoxic medications, no evidence of shock, and no history of kidney disease. There are two types of hepatorenal syndrome and both are usually caused by a precipitating event (infection, bleeding, overdiuresis, and acute hepatitis). Type 1 HRS presents suddenly and progresses quickly, with a creatinine level greater than 2.5 mg/dL in less than 2 weeks. Type 2 HRS progresses slowly with creatinine in the 1.5 to 2.5 mg/dL range (Yadav & Vargas, 2015). Patients with type 1 HRS have a high mortality (80% die within 2 weeks), with only 10% of patients surviving after 3 months. Patients with type 2 HRS have a better survival rate. Patients are more likely to develop HRS with time; 39% of patients with cirrhosis and ascites will develop HRS in 5 years (Wadei, Mai, Ahsan, & Gonwa, 2006).

At the end of this chapter, the reader will be able to:

1. Define hepatorenal syndrome and discuss its causes
2. State treatment options for type 1 HRS
3. State treatment options for type 2 HRS

ASSESSMENT FINDINGS

Patients with HRS may present without symptoms. Others may have acute worsening of liver function (such as worsening jaundice and hepatic encephalopathy), fever, chills, hypotension, tachycardia (signs of sepsis), dry skin and mucous membranes (dehydration and/or over diuresis), dizziness, cold intolerance, or other signs of anemia (if gastrointestinal bleeding is a complication).

PERTINENT LABORATORY FINDINGS

Laboratory testing should include complete blood count, complete metabolic panel, and liver function testing. Usually, HRS is caused by a precipitant, so those causes should be investigated and properly treated. Blood and urine cultures may be required to evaluate for sepsis. Careful monitoring of renal function to reevaluate for improvement or deterioration is essential.

IMAGING STUDIES

A renal ultrasound is usually obtained when there is an acute rise in creatinine to ensure no other etiologies are contributing to the rise in creatinine level, such as kidney stone, chronic renal damage (from diabetes or hypertension), or other issues.

MANAGEMENT

All patients with HRS should discontinue diuretics. If the patient has tense ascites, paracentesis should be performed, with appropriate albumin infusion given to correct volume loss. All possible precipitants for development of HRS should be investigated, including evaluating for sepsis, gastrointestinal bleeding, malnutrition issues, electrolyte imbalances, and acute hepatitis (viral or alcoholic). If precipitants are found, appropriate management should be commenced. The aim of medication management is to improve renal function and maintain survival until liver transplant is possible. Avoidance of nephrotoxic medications/intravenous (IV) contrast dye is necessary. Urgent liver transplant evaluation is suggested. Liver transplant will cure HRS (Runyon, 2013; Wadei et al., 2006; Yadav & Vargas, 2015).

Type 1 HRS

Patients with type 1 HRS require immediate hospitalization to the intensive care unit for management. Central-line placement is necessary to evaluate volume status, which guides providers in knowing how much volume is required (Sola, Guevara, & Gines, 2013; Wadei et al., 2006). Medication management includes administration of albumin, octreotide (200 mcg three times per day) and midodrine (12.5 mg three times per day). Use of vasoactive drugs is needed to increase renal perfusion. In some cases, urgent need for hemodialysis or renal replacement therapy (RRT) may be needed. If hypotension occurs, vasopressors (e.g., terlipressin outside the United States, norepinephrine in the United States) may be necessary to improve mean arterial pressure to greater than 65 mmHg. Consultation with a nephrologist, preferably at a transplant center, is necessary. Urgent liver transplant evaluation is warranted (Runyon, 2013; Wadei et al., 2006; Yadav & Vargas, 2015).

Type 2 HRS

Most patients with type 2 HRS can be managed as outpatients if clinically stable and no other complications arise. Midodrine and octreotide can be used for patients with type 2 HRS. Treatment of refractory ascites is helpful. To control ascites, transjugular intrahepatic portosystemic stent-shunt (TIPS) may be an option for certain patients (see Chapter 22; Runyon, 2013; Sola et al., 2013; Wadei et al., 2006; Yadav & Vargas, 2015).

ICD-10 CODE

Hepatorenal syndrome K76.7

FAST FACTS in a NUTSHELL ════════

- HRS is a condition in which renal failure develops in patients with cirrhosis and ascites. There are two types: type 1 HRS and type 2 HRS.
- Diagnostic criteria include:
  - Creatinine greater than or equal to 1.5 mg/dL
  - No improvement after 2 days of hydration (albumin/volume expanders) with discontinuation of diuretics
  - No recent use of nephrotoxic medications
  - No evidence of shock
  - No history of kidney disease
- HRS is usually caused by a precipitating event (infection, bleeding, overdiuresis, acute hepatitis).
- Goals of treatment of HRS are to preserve renal function and prolong survival until time of liver transplant.
- Liver transplant cures HRS.

REFERENCES

Runyon, B. (2013). Introduction to the revised American Association for the Study of Liver Diseases practice guideline. Management of adult patients with ascites due to cirrhosis: Update 2012. *Hepatology,* 57(4), 1651–1653.

Sola, E., Guevara, M., & Gines, P. (2013). Current treatment strategies for hepatorenal syndrome. *Clinical Liver Disease,* 2(3), 136–139.

Wadei, H. M., Mai, M. L., Ahsan, N., & Gonwa, T. A. (2006). Hepatorenal syndrome: Pathophysiology and management. *Clinical Journal of the American Society of Nephrology,* 1(5), 1066–1079.

Yadav, A., & Vargas, H. E. (2015). Care of the patient with cirrhosis. *Clinical Liver Disease,* 5(4), 100–104.

27

Hepatopulmonary Syndrome

Hepatopulmonary syndrome (HPS) is a condition that affects end-stage liver disease patients in which intra-pulmonary shunting, or pulmonary vascular dilation, causes hypoxemia. Five to 32% of patients with cirrhosis have HPS (Singh & Sager, 2009). HPS has been associated with a higher mortality rate and poor outcomes. Liver transplant can cure this disorder; however, it does take several months to completely resolve hypoxemia. Diagnostic criteria for HPS include (a) evidence of intra-pulmonary shunt (seen on echocardiogram with bubble study), (b) hypoxemia as evidenced by alveolar–arterial (A–a) oxygen gradient greater than or equal to 15 while breathing room air or partial pressure of oxygen less than 80 mmHg, and (c) presence of liver disease with portal hypertension (Hurtado-Cordovi, Lipka, Singh, Shahzad, & Mustacchia, 2011; Iyer, 2014; Singh & Sager, 2009).

At the end of this chapter, the reader will be able to:

1. State the three criteria that must be present to diagnose hepatopulmonary syndrome
2. Identify two physical examination findings that may be present
3. Name three treatment options for management of HPS

ASSESSMENT FINDINGS

The patient with HPS may have very mild symptoms or be asymptomatic, or can the effects be severe, in which case patients require high-flow oxygen continuously to maintain adequate oxygen saturation. Patients may have signs of prolonged hypoxemia, including clubbing, platypnea (dyspnea brought on by sitting upright and improved with lying down), cyanosis, spider nevi, and systolic murmur on physical examination (Iyer, 2014; Singh & Sager, 2009). One of the most common symptoms is dyspnea on exertion (Singh & Sager, 2009).

PERTINENT LABORATORY FINDINGS

Arterial blood gases are obtained on room air, and oxygen saturation levels are evaluated. Routine laboratory data is helpful as well (see Chapter 21).

IMAGING STUDIES

An echocardiogram with bubble (shunt) study is performed to evaluate for an intrapulmonary shunt, which is one of the elements comprising the diagnostic triad of HPS.

MANAGEMENT

Liver transplant is curative for HPS, with most transplant recipients having improvement in oxygenation after 1 year (Lv & Fan, 2015). The United Network for Organ Sharing (UNOS) policy allows for an additional Model for End-Stage Liver Disease (MELD) points to be granted to those individuals who have HPS because of its poor prognosis and the high mortality associated with HPS (Singh & Sager, 2009). When listed with a higher MELD score, the likelihood of transplantation is more probable.

There have been several medical therapies that have been researched to treat HPS, including inhaled nitric oxide, aspirin, pentoxifylline (PTX), methylene blue, and garlic. However, there remains to be no Food and Drug Administration (FDA)-approved medication to medically treat HPS (Lv & Fan, 2015).

ICD 10 CODE

Hepatopulmonary syndrome: K76.81

FAST FACTS in a NUTSHELL

1. HPS has been associated with a high mortality rate and poor outcomes.
2. Diagnostic criteria for HPS includes (a) evidence of intrapulmonary shunt (seen on echocardiogram with bubble study), (b) hypoxemia as evidenced by an A–a oxygen gradient greater than or equal to 15 while breathing room air or partial pressure of oxygen less than 80 mmHg, and (c) presence of liver disease with portal hypertension.
3. Liver transplant can cure this disorder; however, it does take several months to completely resolve hypoxemia.

REFERENCES

Hurtado-Cordovi, J. M., Lipka, S., Singh, J., Shahzad, G., & Mustacchia, P. (2011). Diagnostic challenge of hepatopulmonary syndrome in a patient with coexisting structural heart disease. *Case Reports in Hepatology, 2011*(386709). doi:10.1155/2011/386709

Iyer, V. N. (2014). Liver transplantation for hepatopulmonary syndrome. *Clinical Liver Disease, 4*(2), 38–41.

Lv, Y., & Fan, D. (2015). Hepatopulmonary syndrome. *Digestive Diseases and Sciences, 60,* 1914–1923.

Singh, C., & Sager, J. S. (2009). Pulmonary complications of cirrhosis. *Medical Clinics of North America, 93*(4), 871–883.

28

Hepatocellular Carcinoma

All patients with cirrhosis are at a higher risk for developing hepatocelluar carcinoma (HCC). Other patients at high risk include hepatitis B carriers, patients with a family history of HCC, patients with diabetes or obesity, smokers, males, and those who are infected with HIV (Agarwal, 2012; Yadav & Vargas, 2015). There are over 28,000 new cases of HCC annually, and another 20,000 deaths every year, making it the second most common cause of cancer death worldwide (Goroll & Mulley, 2014; Hickey, Lewandowski, & Salem, 2016).

At the end of this chapter, the reader will be able to:

1. Name two risk factors for the development of HCC
2. Identify how often HCC screening should be performed in patients with HCC
3. Discuss treatment options for HCC management

ASSESSMENT FINDINGS

Patients may be asymptomatic (especially when the patient does not have cirrhosis) or have findings consistent with cirrhosis (see Chapter 21).

PERTINENT LABORATORY FINDINGS

Alpha-fetoprotein is commonly measured in patients at risk for HCC; however, it is a poor marker of disease (Yadav & Vargas, 2015).

IMAGING STUDIES

It is recommended that all patients at high risk for developing HCC be screened by ultrasound every 6 months. To diagnose and treat HCC in its early stages, surveillance is extremely important (Crissien & Frenette, 2014). If ultrasound shows an area of concern for malignancy, further imaging studies are required. Studies have showed that in its early stages HCC is associated with a better prognosis and better patient outcomes than at advanced liver cancer stages (Fitzmorris & Singal, 2015). Options are MRI, CT, or liver biopsy. Diagnostic criteria are identified when arterial enhancement is seen and then are washed out in subsequent images. Liver biopsy is recommended in the patient without cirrhosis or if imaging studies do not reveal classic findings (Yadav & Vargas, 2015).

MANAGEMENT

Patients with HCC are managed by specialists, including a hepatologist and hematologist/oncologist. Surgical treatment options include tumor resection, radiofrequency ablation, or liver transplant (must meet certain tumor criteria to qualify). Other options include chemotherapy, transarterial chemoembolization (TACE), percutaneous ethanol injection, or radioembolization (Crissien & Frenette, 2014; Fitzmorris & Singal, 2015).

Radioembolization can be performed with ^{90}Y, or yttrium-90, allowing for local radiation of HCC tumors (Hickey et al., 2016). This procedure is done in specialized interventional radiology suites.

Sorafenib (Nexavar) is approved by the Food and Drug Administration (FDA) for the medical treatment of advanced stages of liver cancer. Side effects include hypertension, diarrhea, fatigue, lack of appetite, and dermatological complications, including a hand–foot skin reaction. Doses can be adjusted to better tolerate side effects (Granito et al., 2016).

Some patients with HCC may meet certain criteria for a liver transplant. Called *Milan criteria*, these criteria state that the tumor must be a single tumor with a diameter less than or equal to 5 cm, or the patient may have up to three tumors, each with a diameter less than or equal to 3 cm with no extrahepatic involvement and no major vessel involvement (Kim et al., 2010). Because of the poor prognosis and high mortality associated with HCC, the United Network for Organ Sharing (UNOS) policy allows for additional Model for End-Stage Liver Disease (MELD) points to be granted to these individuals, which moves the patient higher on the waiting list (decreasing wait time).

ICD-10 CODE

Liver cell carcinoma: C22.0

FAST FACTS in a NUTSHELL

1. HCC is the second most common cause of cancer death worldwide.
2. In an attempt to diagnose and treat HCC in its early stages, surveillance is extremely important.
3. Patients with HCC are managed by specialists, including a hepatologist and hematologist/oncologist.
4. Treatment options include tumor resection, radiofrequency ablation, or liver transplant (must meet certain tumor criteria to qualify), chemotherapy, transarterial chemoembolization (TACE), percutaneous ethanol injection, or radioembolization.

REFERENCES

Agarwal, P. D. (2012). What primary care providers need to know about hepatocellular carcinoma. *Clinical Liver Disease, 1*(6), 217–219.

Crissien, A. M., & Frenette, C. (2014).Current management of hepatocellular carcinoma. *Gatroenterology and Hepatology, 10*(3), 153–161.

Fitzmorris, P., & Singal, A. K. (2015). Surveillance and diagnosis of hepatocellular carcinoma. *Gastroenterology and Hepatology, 11*(1), 38–46.

Goroll, A. H., & Mulley, A. G. (2014). *Primary care medicine: Office evaluation and management of the adult patient* (7th ed., pp. 459–628). Philadelphia, PA: Lippincott Williams & Wilkins.

Granito, A., Marinelli, S., Negrini, G., Menetti, S., Benevento, F., & Bolondi, L. (2016). Prognostic significance of adverse effects in patients with hepatocellular carcinoma treated with sorafenib. *Therapeutic Advances in Gastroenterology, 9*(2), 240–249.

Hickey, R. M., Lewandowski, R. J., & Salem, R. (2016). Yttrium-90 radioembolization for hepatocellular carcinoma. *Seminars in Nuclear Medicine, 46*(2), 105–108

Kim, J. M., Kwon, C. H., Joh, J. W. Kim, S. J., Shin, M., Kim, E. Y., . . . Lee, S. K. (2010). Patients with unresectable hepatocellular carcinoma beyond Milan criteria: Should we perform transarterial chemoembolization or liver transplantation? *Transplantation Proceedings, 42*(3), 821–824.

Yadav, A., & Vargas, H. E. (2015). Care of the patient with cirrhosis. *Clinical Liver Disease, 5*(4), 100–104.

29

Malnutrition/Vitamin Deficiencies

Malnutrition and vitamin deficiencies are very common in patients with cirrhosis, occurring in over 80% of cases. Some reasons that contribute to this tendency toward malnutrition include inadequate intake; hypermetabolic state; poor production of protein as a result of a damaged liver; increased abdominal girth (ascites) caused by early satiety; the inability to eat desired foods because of fluid, salt, and protein restrictions; socioeconomic obstacles; malabsorption resulting from bacterial overgrowth of the gut; bowel edema from portosystemic shunting; and deficiencies of bile salts (Lalama & Saloum, 2016). Patients with cirrhosis and malnutrition are at higher risk for complications and death, as well as poor wound healing and longer recovery time if they undergo a transplant (Johnson, Overgard, Cohen, & DiBaise, 2013). It is important for providers to understand and recognize malnutrition in this patient population to provide early intervention. An optimal nutrition status improves outcomes for the patient with cirrhosis.

At the end of this chapter, the reader will be able to:

1. Name two contributing causes for the development of malnutrition in the patient with cirrhosis
2. State two methods used to recognize malnutrition in the patient with cirrhosis
3. Discuss optimal protein and calorie recommendations for the patient with cirrhosis

ASSESSMENT FINDINGS

A thorough history should reveal past dietary history, recent weight loss or gain (comparison of the weight change of the past 2 weeks versus the weight change of the past 6 months), change in appetite, nausea, vomiting, diarrhea, loss of appetite, and functional status (ability to perform activities of daily living). Physical examination should note edema or fluid retention, muscle wasting (typically deltoids and triceps), and subcutaneous fat loss. The subjective global assessment (SGA) is a useful tool used to grade the degree of malnutrition by noting the degree of muscle wasting, presence of ascites, weight loss, and other factors. Scores are graded as A (well nourished), B (moderately malnourished), or C (severely malnourished). Anthropomorphic measures that measure midarm circumference and triceps skinfold thickness are recommended. This test should be performed by a provider with experience performing these tests. Another test that can be used is the handgrip strength test, which has been shown to be a predictor of complications in patients with cirrhosis (Lalama & Saloum, 2016).

PERTINENT LABORATORY FINDINGS

Deficiencies, especially of fat-soluble vitamins, are common in patients with cirrhosis. Deficiencies should be noted and corrected with supplementation. Micronutrients that may be deficient in this population include magnesium, thiamine, pyridoxine, zinc, selenium, iron, folic acid, and choline (Johnson et al., 2013).

Laboratory testing to evaluate for malnutrition in patients with cirrhosis can include tests for serum albumin, prealbumin, prothrombin with international normalized ratio [INR], creatinine height index, and immunoglobulin levels (investigating for immune responses). The results of these studies may be abnormal simply because of liver disease and not purely because of malnutrition. Therefore, there is no reliable laboratory marker for malnutrition in the patient with cirrhosis (Montano-Loza, 2014).

IMAGING STUDIES

Dual-energy x-ray absorptiometry (DEXA) and bioelectrical impedance analysis (BIA) are tests that can evaluate for malnutrition. However, these tests are expensive and not readily available. Other possible imaging studies include CT scan to evaluate abdominal muscle mass (Johnson et al., 2013).

MANAGEMENT

It is recommended that all patients with cirrhosis have a nutrition screening for malnutrition. Repeat nutritional assessment should be performed intermittently, every 6 months to 1 year and during acute changes in clinical condition. Caloric intake should be 25 to 40 kcal/kg/day and protein intake should be 1.2 to 1.5 g/kg. Prior treatment recommendations for patients with cirrhosis and hepatic encephalopathy were to restrict protein intake. Latest research supports that protein intake should not be restricted, fasting should be avoided, and branched chain amino acids (BCAAs) may assist in achieving adequate daily protein intake. Enteral feedings may be needed if patients are not able to meet caloric needs with oral intake (Lalama & Saloum, 2016). Patients are encouraged to take small frequent meals and have a bedtime snack (Johnson et al., 2013).

There are several restrictions that may be required for the patient with cirrhosis. In patients with ascites, sodium intake should be restricted to 2 grams per day. Fluid intake may be restricted if serum sodium levels become less than 125 mEq/L (Lalama & Saloum, 2016).

ICD-10 CODE

Other specified nutritional deficiencies: E63.8
Vitamin deficiency, unspecified: E56.9
Vitamin A deficiency, unspecified: E50.9
Vitamin D deficiency, unspecified: E55.9
Deficiency of vitamin K: E56.1
Unspecified protein-calorie malnutrition: E46
Unspecified severe protein-calorie malnutrition: E43
Moderate protein-calorie malnutrition: E44.0

FAST FACTS in a NUTSHELL

1. Malnutrition and vitamin deficiencies are very common in patients with cirrhosis, occurring in over 80% of cases.
2. Factors that contribute to malnutrition include inadequate intake, hypermetabolic state, poor production of protein caused by the damaged liver, early satiety, socioeconomic obstacles, and malabsorption.
3. An optimal nutrition status improves outcomes for the patient with cirrhosis.
4. The SGA is a useful tool used to grade the degree of malnutrition by noting the degree of muscle wasting, presence of ascites, weight loss, and other factors. Scores are graded as A (well nourished), B (moderately malnourished), or C (severely malnourished).
5. Anthropomorphic measures that measure midarm circumference and triceps skin-fold thickness are recommended. This test should be performed by a provider with experience performing such tests.
6. Another test that can be used is the handgrip strength test, which has been shown to be a predictor of complications in patients with cirrhosis.
7. Caloric intake should be 25 to 40 kcal/kg/day and protein intake should be 1.2 to 1.5 g/kg.
8. Patients should not restrict protein intake.

Johnson, T. M., Overgard, E. B., Cohen, A. E., & DiBaise, J. K. (2013). Nutrition assessment and management in advanced liver disease. *Nutrition in Clinical Practice, 28*(1), 15–29.

Lalama, M. A., & Saloum, Y. (2016). Nutrition, fluid, and electrolytes in chronic liver disease. *Clinical Liver Disease, 7*(1), 18–20.

Montano-Loza, A. J. (2014). Clinical relevance of sarcopenia in patients with cirrhosis. *World Journal of Gastroenterology, 20*(25), 8061–8071.

PART
V

Liver Transplantation

30

Transplant Recipient Considerations

Liver transplantation should be discussed in the patient with decompensated cirrhosis who has a Model for End-Stage Liver Disease (MELD) score of 15 or greater. The MELD score is used to determine the severity of liver disease, taking into account the total bilirubin, international normalized ratio (INR), and creatinine levels, as well as whether a patient has developed renal failure requiring dialysis. The new MELD-Na score is now used to prioritize the waiting list for liver transplantation (established by the United Network for Organ Sharing [UNOS]) if the patient's MELD is greater than 11 (Kalra, Wedd, & Biggins, 2016). (See Chapter 21 for further details.) Scores range from 9 to 40, with less than 9 being too early for transplant and 40 indicating an urgent need for transplant. A 3-month survival is estimated, with a MELD of 9 suggesting 90% survival after 3 months, and a score of 40 indicating 7% survival at 3 months (Martin, DiMartini, Feng, Brown, & Fallon, 2014; Wiesner et al., 2003). When caring for patients with cirrhosis, it is help-ful for providers to understand the basic liver transplant evaluation process, as well as long-term postoperative management (see Chapter 32). For contraindications for liver transplant, see Table 30.1.

At the end of this chapter, the reader will be able to:

1. Name two contraindications to liver transplantation
2. Name at least four steps that are involved in the liver transplant evaluation process
3. Discuss patient outcomes after the liver transplant

TABLE 30.1 Contraindications to Liver Transplantation

AIDS	Proven noncompliance
Anatomic abnormalities	Severe cardiac or pulmonary disorders
Malignancy outside the liver	Hepatocellular carcinoma, with metastasis
Alcohol or substance abuse	
Lack of caregiver and/or support system	Fulminant hepatic failure with abnormal intracranial pressure (ICP) > 50 mmHg
MELD < 15	
Active infection/sepsis, uncontrolled	Hemangiosarcoma
	Cholangiocarcinoma, with metastasis

MELD, Model for End-stage Liver Disease.
Source: Martin et al. (2014).

EVALUATION PROCESS

The evaluation process is very thorough. All potential causes of liver disease are investigated. Laboratory testing includes complete blood count, complete metabolic panel, coagulation studies, liver function tests, viral hepatitis serologies, immunologic testing (antinuclear antibody [ANA], antimitochondrial antibody [AMA]), tumor markers (alpha-fetoprotein, Ca 19-9), thyroid function test, cholesterol levels, and drug and alcohol testing. A comprehensive cardiac workup is completed, including electrocardiogram, echocardiogram, stress test, and possible heart catheterization if coronary artery disease has been present or is suspected. Pulmonary function is evaluated by pulmonary function tests, arterial blood gases, and walking oximetry. Malignancy must be ruled out, especially if liver cancer is the indication for transplantation. Radiologic imaging studies include CT scan and possible MRI. Blood flow in and around the liver is examined and evaluated for portal vein thrombosis or other issues that may cause surgery to be difficult. Colonoscopy is performed if a recent test has not been done; endoscopy is performed to evaluate portal hypertension, to rule out varices, or to treat varices with ligation if correctable. If issues come up in the evaluation process that require expert consultation, those consults are requested (Flynn, 2003). For example, in the patient with a long history of chronic obstructive pulmonary disease (COPD), a pulmonary consult would be requested to clear the patient for surgery from a pulmonary standpoint. All patients undergoing evaluation receive consultations from the social work, nutrition, and pharmacy departments. The social worker reviews the patient's financial and caregiver status to ensure that the patient is able to obtain and pay for required posttransplant medications, and that adequate social support and a primary caregiver are available to guide and assist the patient with all needs. Patients may have difficulty understanding key aspects of surgery and/or postoperative processes and medication. It is essential that a primary caregiver is identified to assist with the complex medical regimen.

Once the evaluation process is completed, patients are brought back for a clinic visit to review all results. A multidisciplinary committee reviews all information and jointly decides whether to place the patient on the waiting list for transplant, to deny the patient for transplant, or to defer until further testing is completed. Once listed, patients are allowed to "wait" at home if the distance to the transplant center allows arrival in 4 to 6 hours. The patient is assigned a nurse coordinator who will assist the patient with questions and concerns, adjust schedules, review medications, and provide thorough education on the transplant process.

During the wait time, complications can develop. Complications are recognized and managed. Hospitalizations are frequent, as the longer a patient with decompensated cirrhosis waits for a transplant, the greater the likelihood complications will arise. Patients are told to abide by nutrition guidelines to maintain optimal nutrition. Activity is encouraged, as muscle mass is lost quickly in these patients.

SURGERY, PROGNOSIS, AND OUTCOME

When an organ that is suitable for a patient on the waiting list is identified, the patient is admitted to the hospital. History and physical examination are performed to ensure no new complications have occurred. Laboratory data are obtained, an electrocardiogram and chest radiograph are performed to ensure the heart and lungs are functioning well. The patient should remain NPO (nothing by mouth) for 6 to 12 hours prior to surgery. Blood, anesthesia, and surgical consents are signed. All questions and concerns the patient and caregivers/support system may have are addressed. Typically, surgery lasts from 4 to 8 hours, depending on the patient's prior surgical history and on complications that may arise intraoperatively. Donor organs are characterized as *donation after brain death* (DBD), which is the standard donation with the most optimal outcomes; *donation after cardiac death* (DCD), and *living donor liver transplantation* (LDLT). Split liver transplantations have been performed, but usually are for pediatric patients.

At the time of surgery, the patient is put to sleep by the anesthesia team. The donor liver is prepped in another area on the "back table" and is examined to ensure suitability for transplantation. The surgeon removes the donor gallbladder. Surgery is begun by making bilateral subcostal incisions along the abdomen as an "upside down Y" or "Mercedes" fashion. Efforts are made to perform the hepatectomy, or removing the diseased liver. This can be difficult if the patient is very coagulopathic or has had prior abdominal infections or surgeries that have caused adhesions. Once hemostasis is achieved, the donor liver can be placed in the recipient. Vessels are reconnected, including the donor suprahepatic vena cava to the recipient inferior vena cava (IVC), the donor to the recipient portal veins, and the connection of the hepatic arteries and bile ducts. If possible, a biliary tube is placed within the biliary anastomosis, also called *duct-to-duct anastomosis* or *choledochocholedochostomy*. If the patient had diseased bile ducts, such as in primary sclerosing cholangitis or primary biliary cirrhosis, the donor bile duct is usually connected to the recipient's small bowel. This is called a *Roux-en-Y anastomosis*, or *Roux-en-Y choledochojejunostomy*. After all connections are made and the abdomen is investigated for bleeding, leaks, and removal of surgical instruments and sponges, the abdomen is sutured closed. Sometimes abdominal drains, or Jackson–Pratt drains, are placed to allow for drainage of fluid. Staples are placed along the incision to close the skin (Flynn, 2003).

Immediate complications that can occur include bleeding, respiratory failure (unable to arouse from anesthesia), pain issues, and acute kidney failure (even if renal issues were not a problem prior to transplant). For further postoperative information, see Chapter 32.

Survival after a liver transplant is better now than ever before. With improved immunosuppression and more transplant centers with extensive experience, patients who once were expected to live for 3 months can now be expected to live another 10 years. The 5-year overall graft (liver) survival was 70.2% for those patients who received a liver transplant in 2009. Patients who received a DCD graft; older patients (than age 65); or those patients who had a re-transplant, HCV, or HCC had poorer outcomes than other patients without these issues (Kim et al., 2016).

ICD-10 CODE

Liver transplant: Z94.4

========================= *FAST FACTS in a NUTSHELL*

1. There are several contraindications to receiving a liver transplant, including sepsis/uncontrolled infection, low MELD score, active alcohol or substance abuse, or metastatic malignancy.
2. The liver transplant evaluation process is very thorough; it investigates all body systems to ensure best patient outcomes and proper organ allocation.
3. Social support is a huge factor in ensuring good patient outcomes and patient survival.
4. If complications arise while the patient is waiting for transplant, issues are treated appropriately. If acute infection occurs, the patient is placed off the waiting list until infection is controlled.
5. Survival after liver transplant is better now than ever before.

REFERENCES

Flynn, B. M. (2003). Liver transplantation. In S. A. Cupples & L. Ohler (Eds.), *Transplantation nursing secrets: Questions and answers reveal the secrets to successful transplantation nursing.* Philadelphia, PA: Hanley & Belfus.

Kalra, A., Wedd, J. P., & Biggins, S. W. (2016). Changing prioritization for transplantation: MELD-Na, hepatocellular carcinoma exceptions, and more. *Current Opinion in Organ Transplantation, 21*(2), 120–126.

Kim, W. R., Lake, J. R., Smith, J. M., Skeans, M. A., Schladt, D. P., Edwards, . . . Kasiske, B. L. (2016). Liver. *American Journal of Transplantation, 16*(S2), 69–98. doi:10.1111/ajt.13668

Martin, P., DiMartini, A., Feng, S., Brown, R., & Fallon, M. (2014). Evaluation for liver transplantation in adults: 2013 Practice guideline by the AASLD and the American Society of Transplantation. *Hepatology, 59*(3), 1144–1165.

Wiesner, R., Edwards, E., Freeman, R., Harper, A., Kim, R., Kamath, P., . . . United Network for Organ Sharing Liver Disease Severity Score Committee. (2003). Model for end-stage liver disease (MELD) and allocation of donor livers. *Gastroenterology, 124*(1), 91–96.

3 |

Transplant Donor Considerations

Live donor liver transplantation (LDLT) is an option for liver transplantation. In an effort to reduce wait time for some patients needing a transplant, and in an effort to increase the number of donors available, LDLTs were instituted as a possible alternative to the standard brain-death donor. LDLT was initially only performed for pediatric patients (Flynn, 2003); however, it has become increasingly popular for adult liver transplant and will continue to be popular as surgical techniques are refined. A left lateral segmentectomy (donation of the left lobe) has proved to have a lower risk of complications than a right lobectomy (Anderson-Shaw & Cotler, 2015).

At the end of this chapter, the reader will be able to:

1. Name two reasons why a living liver donor may not qualify for donation
2. Discuss the recipient outcomes of living liver donation
3. Discuss the donor outcomes of living liver donation

SELECTION OF AN ACCEPTABLE LIVING LIVER DONOR

Like any surgery, the living liver donor must be aware of all risks associated with the procedure, and the decision to donate must be completely noncoerced and self-directed. These individuals are usually in good health, aged between 21 and 55, with little to no comorbidities (uncontrolled diabetes or hypertension, coronary artery disease, etc.). Surgical expert consultation should review radiological imaging to ensure that anatomy is acceptable for living liver donation. A thorough evaluation, similar to the exam given to the transplant recipient, is required. United Network for Organ Sharing (UNOS) recommends an independent donor advocate evaluate the donor as well. Patients should not be coerced into surgery in any way, and psychosocial consultation is recommended to fully evaluate the patient for the reason for donation (Brown, 2008).

DONOR OUTCOMES

Worldwide, the donor mortality is 0.15%. Complications include biliary complications (bile leak and/or strictures), pneumonia, incisional hernia, wound infections, or small bowel obstruction. Complications occur in approximately 10% of cases. The quality of life for patients who have donated a liver has been investigated. Most patients report that they would donate again, even if donor complications did occur (Brown, 2008). Liver regeneration does occur post donation, with most donors having a near-complete recovery after 1 year (Cotler, 2015).

RECIPIENT OUTCOMES

One meta-analysis by Wan, Yu, and Xia (2014) compared operative outcomes of deceased donor liver transplant (DDLT) and LDLT recipients. LDLT patients had a longer surgery time and a shorter cold ischemic time (time of graft outside of body without blood supply). LDLT patients also had more instances of complications, including biliary complications, vascular complications, and even re-transplantation. It has been argued that with more experience in performing LDLT, the rate of complications will decrease (Wan et al., 2014).

ICD-10 CODE

Liver donor: Z52.6

=== FAST FACTS in a NUTSHELL

1. Living liver donation transplantation is an option for liver transplant recipients.
2. The living liver donor must be aware of all risks associated with the procedure, and the decision to donate must be completely noncoerced and self-directed.
3. These individuals are usually in good health, aged between 21 and 55, with little to no comorbidities (uncontrolled diabetes or hypertension, coronary artery disease, etc.).
4. Significant complications can occur after living liver donation.

REFERENCES

Anderson-Shaw, L., & Cotler, S. J. (2015). Ethical issues in liver transplantation. Retrieved from www.uptodate.com/contents/ethical-issues-in-liver-transplantation?source=search_result&search=Ethical+issues+in+liver&selectedTitle=1%7E150.html

Brown, R. S. (2008). Liver donors in liver transplantation. *Gastroenterology, 134*(6), 1802–1813. doi:10.1053/j.gastro.2008.02.092

Cotler, S. J. (2015). Living donor liver transplantation. Retrieved from www.uptodate.com/contents/living-donor-liver-transplantation?source=search_result&search=Living+donor+liver+transplantation.&selectedTitle=1%7E23.html

Flynn, B. M. (2003). Liver transplantation. In S. A. Cupples & L. Ohler (Eds.), *Transplantation nursing secrets: Questions and answers reveal the secrets to successful transplantation nursing.* (pp. 151–171). Philadelphia, PA: Hanley & Belfus.

Wan, P., Yu, X., & Xia, Q. (2014). Operative outcomes of adult living donor liver transplantation and deceased donor liver transplantation: A systematic review and meta-analysis. *Liver Transplantation, 20*(4), 425–436. doi:10.1002/lt.23836

32

Posttransplant Care

For patients suffering from end-stage liver disease, liver transplantation is seen as a cure and a new chance of life. In the first few months after liver transplantation, medical care is managed by the transplant center and the specialists who performed the transplant surgery. Thereafter, medical care is directed by the patient's primary care provider, unless there are concerns regarding liver transplant complications. Any issues regarding changes in immunosuppression, infection, organ rejection, recurrent liver disease, or renal issues should be managed by a transplant center (preferably where the patient had the surgery). Providers should be aware of long-term care recommendations for the transplant patient after surgery to ensure optimal health for these individuals.

At the end of this chapter, the reader will be able to:

1. Name three routine screening tests that should be performed in primary care for the posttransplant patient
2. State two common long-term complications that occur after liver transplant
3. Name one immunosuppressant medication that the posttransplant patient will be on indefinitely

195

PREVENTATIVE MEDICINE

At every primary care visit, providers should discuss with the patient current medications and any recent changes to medications. Certain medications can put the patient at more risk for infection (immunosuppressants), or cause certain side effects, including hypertension, diabetes, and hyperlipidemia (see Table 32.1 for a list of common posttransplant medications). A careful review of comorbidities prior to the transplant and since the transplant is important (Gaglio & Cotler, 2016). Patients should be screened at regular intervals for hypertension, diabetes, hyperlipidemia, renal issues, and bone loss (see Table 32.2 for screening recommendations). Patients should receive regular immunizations, including an annual influenza vaccine, pneumococcal vaccine every 5 years, and hepatitis A and B if not already vaccinated. Routine recommendations for all patients, transplanted or not, include dietary modifications if overweight or obese and encouragement to engage in a routine exercise program. All patients should abstain from alcohol and smoking. For basic aches and pains, patients can take acetaminophen (Tylenol) in lower doses (2 to 3 g per day). All nonsteroidal anti-inflammatory drugs (NSAIDs) should be avoided, as interaction with calcineurin inhibitors (CNIs) can contribute to renal injury.

Because transplant patients are immunosuppressed, several self-protection measures should be taken posttransplant. Patients should perform frequent hand washing and avoid contact with sick individuals. Crowds should be avoided. Sun exposure should be limited, sunscreen should be worn, and clothing should cover exposed skin to minimize exposure. Patients should cook meat to safe temperatures, avoid raw or uncooked/unpasteurized foods, and avoid consuming water from rivers and lakes or water that has not been filtered/purified. Pregnancy is possible posttransplant; however, it should be delayed until 1 year after surgery. Certain immunosuppressant medication (e.g., mycophenalatemofetil) can cause birth defects (Lucey et al., 2013). Patients should be advised regarding contraception options and, if pregnancy is desired, a detailed, informed discussion should occur among the patient's gynecologist/obstetrician, hepatologist, and primary care provider.

TABLE 32.1 Common Posttransplant Medications

Drug	Approximate Cost	Length of Treatment
Immunosuppressants		
Tacrolimus (Prograf)	$130/month	Indefinitely*
Cyclosporine (Gengraf or Neoral)	$80/month	Indefinitely*
Mycophenalatemofetil (CellCept or Myfortic)	$30/month	3–4 months' posttransplant
Sirolimus (Rapamune)	$200 to 300/month	Indefinitely*
Prednisone (Deltasone)	$10/month	Differs per transplant center 4 months–indefinitely
Everolimus (Zortress)	$900/month	Indefinitely* (sometimes in combination with tacrolimus)
Antiviral Prophylaxis		
Acyclovir (Zovirax—low risk for CMV infection)	$15/month	30 days' posttransplant
or		90 days' posttransplant
Valganciclovir (Valcyte—high risk for CMV infection)	$3,000/month	
Antifungal Prophlaxis		
Nystatin swish and swallow	$20/month	30 days' posttransplant
or		
Clotrimazole (Mycelex Troches)	$150/month	
PJP Prophylaxis		
Sulfamethoxazole/ Trimethoprim (Bactrim)	$10/month	6 months' posttransplant
or	$50–100/month	
Pentamidine (if allergy to sulfa)		
Diabetes/Hyperglycemia		If not diabetic prior to transplant, likely will resolve after 4 months when off steroids
Levemir—$300/month	$300/month	
Novolog—$300/month	$300/month	
Antihypertensives		
Metoprolol (Lopressor)	$10/month	3–4 months to indefinitely

*Patient are usually on prograf OR cyclosporine OR rapamune - not all three at the same time.
PJP, *Pneumocystis jiroveci* pneumonia.

TABLE 32.2 Preventative Screening Recommendations

Annual history and physical examination with PCP	Stress test every 5 years
Dental assessment and cleaning twice a year	Urinalysis, microalbumin, protein every 2–3 months until the first year, then every 6 months
Blood pressure screening every 6 months	Bone mineral density testing every other year
Blood sugar screening every 6 months	Annual PSA (men)
Annual fasting lipid panel (screen for hyperlipidemia)	Annual mammography and Pap smear (women)
Colonoscopy	Dermatologist/full skin evaluation annually for the first 5 years
HCC screening with imaging every 6–12 months	

HCC, hepatocellular carcinoma; PCP, primary care provider; PSA, prostate-specific antigen.

COMMON MEDICAL PROBLEMS AFTER A LIVER TRANSPLANT

Hypertension/Cardiac Issues

Hypertension is one of the most common long-term complications that arise after a liver transplant, occurs in 55% to 85% of patients. The blood pressure goal should be less than 130/80 mmHg. Lifestyle modifications may be needed to gain control of blood pressure, including diet changes and incorporating regular exercise daily. Initially, diuretics and beta blockers are helpful while in hospital. In patients without diabetes or renal issues, amlodipine or nifedipine are options. Some calcium-channel blockers have drug-to-drug interactions with immunosuppressants (e.g., CNIs; Chaney, 2015). First-line agents for the long-term management of patients with diabetes and chronic kidney disease are angiotensin-converting enzyme (ACE) inhibitors or angiotensin receptor blockers (ARBs; Lucey et al., 2013). For patients with low risk of gastrointestinal bleeding and aged between 45 and 79, it would be reasonable to start aspirin daily 4 to 6 months after surgery to minimize cardiovascular risk (Chaney, 2015).

Hyperlipidemia

Initial management includes lifestyle changes and dietary modifications. Weight loss will help if patient is overweight or obese. Omega-3 fatty acid supplementation is recommended for patients with hypertriglyceridemia (without other lipid elevations; Lucey et al., 2013).

Diabetes/Hyperglycemia

Because of the need for high-dose steroids after transplant to reduce the likelihood of organ rejection, hyperglycemia is a common occurrence. The goal in management of posttransplant diabetes is to have hemoglobin A1c less than 7.0%. It is recommended that the patient be provided with education on diabetes and proper dietary/lifestyle changes to help keep blood sugar in an optimal range. Insulin is most commonly given for uncontrolled blood sugars/diabetes. After recovery from the transplant surgery, it is reasonable to consider converting from insulin to oral hypoglycemic agents to control blood sugars (Lucey et al., 2013). It is recommended that patients be in communication with the transplant center regarding any medication changes.

Infection Issues

This patient population is at high risk for infection, with 80% of liver transplant patients developing an infection in the first year (Chaney, 2015). There are several preventive medications these patients take posttransplant to prevent infections (see Table 32.1). Referral to the patient's transplant center and/or hepatologist is recommended in the event of an infection.

Renal Issues

After a liver transplant, patients are at higher risk for developing renal dysfunction. Routine assessment of renal function is recommended at least once per year with urinalysis and urine protein quantification (Lucey et al., 2013). If renal issues arise, immunosuppression usually is adjusted. This should be done at the discretion of the patient's hepatologist/transplant center.

Osteopenia/Osteoporosis

Patients who have had a liver transplant have a higher risk of bone loss. This is thought to occur because of malnutrition, vitamin deficiencies, and long-term steroid use. Patients should have vitamin D levels (25-hydroxy-vitamin D) drawn, and, if low, supplementation should be given. Patients with osteopenia should be placed on calcium with vitamin D for maintenance therapy and should perform regular weight-bearing exercises to reduce further bone loss. Patients may be given bisphosphonate medications if osteoporosis is present or if fractures have occurred (Lucey et al., 2013). Endocrinology consultation is helpful to guide optimal therapy.

Gout

Another side effect of CNIs (e.g., tacrolimus, cyclosporine) is increased uric acid levels, which can contribute to an acute gout attack. For initial management, patients are given colchicine and corticosteroids. Long term management includes the use of allopurinol. However, there is a drug-to-drug interaction with azathioprine resulting in reduced immunosuppression, so cautious use is recommended (Gaglio & Cotler, 2016).

ICD-10 CODE

Aftercare liver transplant: Z48.23
Hypertension: I10.0

Hyperlipidemia: E78.5
Steroid induced hyperglycemia/diabetes: E09.9
Immunosuppressed state: D84.9
Acute kidney failure, unspecified: N17.9
Chronic kidney disease, unspecified: N18.9
Osteopenia: M85.8
Osteoporosis: M81.0
Gout, unspecified site: M10.00

===== *FAST FACTS in a NUTSHELL*

1. Providers should be aware of long-term care recommendations for the posttransplant patient to ensure optimal health for these individuals.
2. Patients should be screened at regular intervals for hypertension, diabetes, hyperlipidemia, renal issues, and bone loss.
3. Patients should receive regular immunizations, including influenza annually, pneumococcal every 5 years, and hepatitis A and B if not already vaccinated.
4. Routine recommendations for all patients, transplanted or not, include dietary modifications if overweight or obese and encouragement to follow a routine exercise program.
5. All patients should abstain from alcohol and smoking.
6. Common long-term complications include hypertension, diabetes, infection, hyperlipidemia, and renal issues.

REFERENCES

Chaney, A. (2015). Primary care management of the liver transplant patient. *Nurse Practitioner, 39*(12), 27–33.

Gaglio, P. J., & Cotler, S. J. (2016). Liver transplantation in adults: Long-term management of transplant recipients. Retrieved from www.uptodate.com/contents/liver-transplantation-in-adults-long-term-management-of-transplant-recipients?source=search_resul

t&search=Liver+transplantation+in+adults&selectedTitle=2%7E
150#H154136866.html

Lucey, M. R., Terrault, N., Ojo, L., Hay, J. E., Neuberger, J., Blumberg, E., & Teperman, L. W. (2013). Long-term management of the successful adult liver transplant: 2012 practice guideline by AASLD and the American Society of Transplantation. *Liver Transplantation, 19*(1), 3–26. doi:10.1002/lt.23566

Index